THAT YOUR FAITH MAY NOT FAIL

Peter's Sermon

by SELAH HELMS

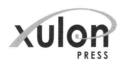

Copyright © 2015 by Selah Helms

That Your Faith May Not Fail
Peter's Sermon
by Selah Helms

Printed in the United States of America.

ISBN 9781498445719

All rights reserved solely by the author. The author guarantees all contents are original and do not infringe upon the legal rights of any other person or work. No part of this book may be reproduced in any form without the permission of the author. The views expressed in this book are not necessarily those of the publisher.

Unless otherwise indicated, Scripture quotations taken from the English Standard Version (ESV). Copyright © 2001 by Crossway, a publishing ministry of Good News Publishers. Used by permission. All rights reserved.

www.xulonpress.com

This book is dedicated to my pastor and husband, Doug Helms—there's no place I'd rather be, through life's joys and sorrows, than alongside him —and to my youngest son, Peter, who has been called to the task of suffering

Acknowledgements

My dear friend Jane has dubbed it "the river of grace" that runs through our home. This book and indeed, the story itself, could not have been told without help from a multitude of people who have come and gone from our front door.

Below is a partial list.

Thank you to all of God's dear people who have with weeping and love prayed us through this journey.

Thanks to Whitney, Rhonda, and Bob and Rita for the green juice that has kept me going over the months when I have been sluggish and wimpy.

Thanks to Miriam, my homeschool mom and RN friend who arrived at seven o'clock every morning for weeks at the hospital, to allow Doug to take time off to get breakfast and coffee after he'd been there all night and to allow me extra time before I had to be there.

Thanks to Jane, Baker, Jeremy, and Nathan H., for helping us get a room ready for Peter when it was time to bring him home.

Thanks to my dear cleaning ladies, who, without judging my dusty corners and happily, scrub my toilets and mop my floor every week, rotating in teams that arrive once a month: Brenda,

Cathy, Melanie, Faye, Sarah, Joan, Carole, and before that, Marty, Melinda, Penny, Sally, and Christy.

Thank you to the nine young men from our church who jumped in on a steep learning curve to install wood floors in our living room after our house took on water and our carpet was ruined. Thanks to the Rock Creek team of men and women who arrived to help us "mop up" after the damage.

Thanks to Therese, who for over a year, sent me almost weekly cards of encouragement and Scripture. Thanks also, for designing and printing Beth's wedding invitations.

Thank you to the individuals and families that sacrificed a week of their time over the past two years to give us some respite time: the McBrides, the Sommers, (two of Peter's speech and debate friends), Rachael (a young nurse from Union University who donated her spring break to Peter's care), and Betsy (the wife of one of Andrew's former and favorite professors).

Thanks to our therapists who have come alongside, to help educate us on all we can do for Peter: Chris, Craig, Megan, Christy B., Jamie, Kamie, Kristin, Rachel, Christy J., and others.

Thanks to all of Mary Ellen's Bible study ladies, who decluttered and reorganized my garage, painted my master bathroom, planted a bounty of fall color in my front beds, and left a freezer full of meals—all in one Tuesday morning.

Thanks to our "dream team" of home healthcare nurses, who've all contributed to keeping Peter healthy and strong: Cassie, Gerard, Angelle, Salvador, Daniel, Nathan B., and Robbie. Thanks to Zeb and Allie, who have been in on this effort behind the scenes.

Thanks to the eleven or twelve dear people who donated enough for us to buy Peter a custom-made wheelchair van, tall enough to fit his 6'4" frame comfortably.

Acknowledgements

Thanks to the busy families that have been willing to donate an hour a week to help with Peter's daily mat sessions: the Kirks and Kevin, Nita, Joe and Jake, Will, Rosemary, the Lusks, the Hughes, Elaine, Kathy, Michal and Brookin, and newly, the McGaughs. The Lord will reward you for your investment in Pete's life and health.

Thanks to those who have run errands and dropped by to spend time with Peter: Michal, Melinda and Daniel, and Rosemary. Thanks to Lennie B for all the laundry detergent and dishwasher soap. Thanks, Betsy, for the Sunday meals.

Thanks to Melanie, a homeschool mom and osteopathic doctor, who between trips to Washington to fight for a privatized approach to medicine, adjusts Peter's bones, muscles, and joints.

Thanks to Susan and Blaine for giving us a week's lodging in Maui and Kauai to celebrate our twenty-ninth wedding anniversary and enjoy some needed rest and recreation time apart from the heavy duties of being a caregiver. Thanks, also, you two, for giving me a bedroom in your house for three days almost every month to have time away to think, renew, and write.

Thanks to the ones who took the time to pore carefully over Pete's book and give valuable feedback: Jane R., Jane H., Becky, Doug, and Susan.

Thanks to Rosemary for singing to Peter, playing her violin for him, doing hours of speech therapy with him, and weeping with us when we weep.

Thank you to my dear friend Jane, who has shared precious memories of Peter's growing up alongside her kids and who weeps with me when I weep and speaks comforting truth into my ears.

Thanks to Gramma and Grampa Helms, for selling their house in Weatherford to move within a mile of us, so that Gramma could be on hand to help with Peter three mornings a week. Gramma has been a constant source of encouragement to us and to Peter and has never stopped believing in God's work in and through Peter's life. She has persevered throughout hours of therapy with greatly varying responses on Peter's part, never giving up hope.

Thank you to my kids Andrew and AmyRose, Joshua and Beth, and Caleb and Hope, for their unflagging support of Peter and for the time they have lovingly and loyally invested in his care, Andrew for giving up a year and two summers of life, and Beth, for not ever complaining about the six plus years it has taken to finish college because of a willing sacrifice on little brother's behalf. Thanks to AmyRose for getting in his face and laughing with him. Thanks to each for trusting God along with their parents, even when it has been a staggering spiritual battle. Thank you for continuing to include Peter in your lives even when it is hard. You have the marks of grace in your hearts.

Thanks most to our Lord Jesus Christ, who has kept us fully dependent on him in a very day-to-day walk, providing only what we need in the moment, through a host of his people, so that we will not be able to depend on any single or few persons, but only to look daily to him. His work makes his people very dear to us.

Truly it has been a river of overflowing grace.

To protect the privacy of the individuals, some names have been changed.

Foreword

In 2005, when Michael Schiavo briefed the media regarding the court order to remove the feeding tube from his minimally conscious wife, Terri, he defended his decision by saying that since her injury, his wife's "biography was over" — she had no more contribution to make in this life. So her feeding tube was removed and she was slowly starved to death over several days' time.

Doug and I followed this story in the news with alarm, but never imagining that some years later our youngest son would sustain the same kind of injury and subsequent disability as did this woman Terri. Watching clips then, the apparent setback to the pro-life cause appalled us. As a pastor's family, we had supported pro-life ministries over the years, including local pregnancy help centers and awareness emphases in the churches where we had served. We saw our country's ethic of life eroding.

Recently, we watched a documentary on the life of Terri Schindler Schiavo. As we reviewed footage we'd seen years ago, we couldn't help but see striking similarities between her condition and that of our son. On July 29, 2010, days before he was to go off to college, Peter suffered a traumatic brain injury in a horrific car accident. The difference, of course, which we hope will become apparent to you as you read this book, is that Peter's life is still valuable to his caregivers, to his family, to his friends, and to many others. Though Terri's parents still valued her life and went through heroic measures to save her, in the end, those in charge of her medical decisions chose not to respect the sanctity of her precious life.

This little epistle, written from the halls of suffering, cries out that our son Peter's biography is not over. He is still making a contribution. His life still has meaning and purpose and dignity.

My ambitions in briefly sketching his life are legion. I want my dear readers to love heaven more. I hope to inspire enough of a vision of heaven that you would be fortified to walk gracefully through the heaviest trial the Lord may send you. I hope to help stock my readers with the theology to face suffering with faith and courage.

I hope that you will want to love your families more, that parents will be inspired to invest more for the kingdom in the lives of their children, and that you will set your face like flint against the distractions that would entangle. I yearn for Christian fathers to devote themselves to regular family devotions, building the Word of life into their children's hearts and minds, and for Christian mothers to consider no opportunity to be greater than the privilege of rearing sons and daughters for Christ.

I also long to attach your heartstrings more fiercely to your church families, on whom you will depend during times of suffering. You will need them. Without this strong attachment, faux believers leave the faith during times of suffering and loss. Their alternatives are despair, bitterness, and medication. Pour your heart and life into your local church. You also need to be sensitive to those Christians around you who are engaged in pitched battle for their faith during times of suffering. Leave off selfish pursuits in order to form the kind of ties with them that will brace their wobbling knees.

My son Andrew warned me of the tendency of authors of biography to indulge in a kind of hagiographic romanticizing of their subjects. Everything I have written here is true and verifiable, but I will still issue a disclaimer that Peter and his family members are sinners and still in the process of working out their salvation in many areas. However, Proverbs tells us that it is possible for a wise son to bring much joy to his parents, and when Peter could walk and talk, he showed himself to be a young man walking humbly with his God. He brought his parents much joy. I hope that Peter's life will inspire other young people to walk in "the Way."

I also desire to raise awareness of Christian classical education. I hope to stir up ideas in the minds of young Christian artists and musicians and writers to take ground in the humanities for the Lordship of Christ. I want to reveal choice vignettes of those Christians who've gone before us, who've contributed great things to the culture and thought life of the world. Their histories will enrich and aid us in following Christ in our own difficulties.

I desire that Peter's life will reveal the beauty of the Lord. I hope that when you read this book, his beauty will be so apparent that you will consider him worthy of giving him your life. I hope you will consider him worthy of anything you must bear in this life. Some are called on to bear the burden of a disabled family member, some to persevere in a difficult marriage, some to strain the limits of their Christian virtue in hostile work or school settings. The Lord has us all in our various boxes that we dare not escape by unrighteous means. As he hedges us into our walls of suffering, we learn obedience by meekness and submission. Peter and we are learning, by the death of Peter's hopes and dreams in this life, to make the Lord our happiness, to yearn for our future lives with him. I hope that he will become your life.

In him, our lives are sacred.

Chapter One

The world is indeed full of peril, and in it there are many dark places, but still there is much that is fair, and though in all lands love is mingled with grief, it grows perhaps the greater. —J.R.R. Tolkien

Peter's dad and I always thought he would make a preacher. Not only was he bright and biblical, but he had an understanding way of coming alongside a person and gently walking them through their thoughts to where they needed to end up.

I remember how, at age eight, Beth came to me in tears of consternation that her six-year-old brother knew more about the doctrines of salvation than she did, and that she had had to submit to his childlike explanation of them to her. As she came to me, grudgingly admitting he knew so much more than she, Peter smiled quietly in the background, waiting for her to return and rejoin their play, unaware of the humiliation he had caused his older sister.

During family movie nights, we noticed that Peter watched movies with an adult's understanding of human nature and a Dickensian warmth of sympathy for men's foibles. We would think he wasn't really paying attention, because he would be spread eagled on the floor on his stomach drawing pictures. But his active mind absorbed everything. He would glance up when a character, completely oblivious, stumbled into some self-created havoc. Then Pete would give a knowing chuckle. Doug and I would meet each other's amazed eye: "He actually caught that!" It was a regular occurrence.

As he grew older, I often gleaned the benefit of Peter's understanding temper. So many times, when I was in a "tizzy," facing my thousand duties of a day between homeschooling and Doug's pastorate, I became bossy and snappish. Peter would walk across the kitchen where I was frantically working and put his arm around me, a kindly twinkle in his eye: "You need some help, Mom? Here, let me help you get supper," — he doubtless believing that his raw display of forbearance was guaranteed to turn the tables on my selfish thoughts. And I have to admit, unconditional love works wonders on a harried mom.

When Pete hit about six feet tall, younger kids at church would sit beside him during the service, copying his sermon notes onto their bulletins. As soon as the last prayer was over, they would beg him to go outside and play with them. Peter would smilingly oblige, waiting until they were content before quietly bowing out to spend time with his peers. When he turned sixteen, in a desire to be more intentional in encouraging his friends in Christ, he began leading a discussion among the teenaged guys on *Don't Waste Your Life* by John Piper.

His hero and oldest brother, Andrew, had gone off to college at Union University when Peter was eleven. From home, Pete watched his older brother navigate the waters of independent living, deciding on which values of his parents to keep, getting to know girls, and planning out his life. My scholarly eldest son periodically went through doldrums of melancholy during those

Chapter One

years, his introvertish temperament besting him at times. On our visits to see him, Peter trotted eagerly across campus, meeting Andrew's friends and professors, piling his boy's plate full of the cafeteria food that Andrew despised, and beating Andrew's roommates at chess. They called Pete "Mini-Helms." He never ceased to admire his academic brother, even while teasing him out of his dark thoughts. One of his New Year's resolutions during those years was to write Andrew encouraging emails.

Together, all of us back home took note when our second son—Caleb, more sociable and rambunctious—arrived at Union. Andrew's freshman year, we all claimed, was marked by phone calls from home, during which his family members encouraged him: "Andrew, get out of your room. You need to be around people sometimes. The books can wait." Caleb's freshman year, on the other hand, inspired family phone calls like, "Caleb, you need to stay in your room. You do have to get your homework done, you know. You will still have time for friends." When our family visited campus, we laughed at stories of how surprised all their Union peers were to find out that Andrew and Caleb Helms were actually brothers.

When Andrew made it into the PhD program at Notre Dame University, the whole family rejoiced. First semester, Andrew would be studying under his long-time hero, Alvin Plantinga. He had made the cut of thirteen students out of hundreds of applicants. Notre Dame was the Christian philosopher's mecca. However, the course load was challenging for Andrew, who had been accustomed to being a big, bespectacled fish in a smaller academic pond at Union University and Texas A&M, where he'd earned his master's degree. Now the "pond" stocked many fish that Andrew viewed as intellectually far superior to him. He had a hard year.

Peter shot off a saucy email to Andrew that fall, with a reference to a family in Fort Worth whose oldest son became a friend of Andrew's at Notre Dame. Of course, it was calculated to "help" him:

Hey Andrew, how are you doing? I'm doing fine thanks for asking. How is the transition into Notre Dame going? I heard that you helped Jeremy Nelson move in on Sunday. On Tuesday, Micah Nelson said I looked just like you. I was like "Puleaze! I'm already having a bad day." Just kidding. Actually, what I really said was, "What a lucky dog that Andrew is."

I heard you went to the CRC church on Sunday. We're still praying that you're able to find a good church (with a nice old male pastor). Too bad you didn't get to meet Dr. Al [Plantinga]. Maybe next time. Have classes started up yet? We all miss you a lot. Any initial weird things or thoughts that have come upon you yet from your new surroundings?

Respond at your convenience.
Your bother,
Peter

Hey Peter, good to hear from you! I'm doing great; glad to hear that you are doing fine and relieved that you still look like me. How's the detective story coming along? You will have to forward it to me when it's done. This past Sunday I went to a church close by. I didn't get to meet the pastor since he was out of town, but one of my fellow philosophy PhD students from ND preached out of the book of Acts (none of your snide comments about philosophers preaching). . . . I have met Dr. Al now, and submitted a short paper to him today; he calls them 'non-papers' so that students will feel less intimidated by the workload in the class. I'm not

Chapter One

sure that it has the desired effect, but we do try to humor him. I will try to write more when I get the chance but send a note any time you feel like it.

Your "bother,"
Andrew

So it was quite within Peter's character that May, to want to swing up through South Bend in order to "cheer Andrew up" on our way to Virginia Beach. At seventeen, Peter had just graduated from our homeschool high school, rattled off his Rachmaninoff and Brahms pieces in the spring recital, and qualified in his speech and debate competitions for the national level of competition for homeschoolers, to be held at a private college in Virginia Beach in early June. He and I would travel there together. Then he would compete in the Lincoln-Douglas debate event, impromptu oratory, and persuasive speaking. In his ten-minute persuasive speech delivered from memory on the topic of Demographic Winter, Peter argued that Christians should enter into childrearing with joy, zeal, and vision.

Peter and I discussed our mission during the eighteen-hour drive to South Bend. We would swing up to spend a week with Andrew, though it was a bit out of the way from our second destination, Virginia Beach, where we would spend a second week. Peter didn't plan to study for his debates as much as he probably should have; he was just happy to have made the cut to the national competition. Instead, he wanted to take time to bless his brother. It was a decision that I came to believe was from the Lord.

"Okay, mom, I'll play some chess with him when he takes study breaks."

"Sounds good," I replied. "While you do that, I'll clean his room and catch him up on his laundry."

"I'll loosen him up, mom. I'll get him to laugh. And maybe I can get him to take me to campus and we can play some racquetball in the gym."

"Then, we can both work on getting some decent meals in his freezer."

"Let's try to make a big meal and have some of his friends over from church or something. Maybe we can stir up his social life."

Together, we sketched out a rough plan for how we could bring some order to the bedroom we'd seen in the background of our Skype visits with Andrew from our home in Fort Worth. We also planned ways we could provide Andrew with lots of creative recreation time.

When we left home after church that day, we packed the car with all kinds of activities that geeky homeschoolers enjoy. Peter chose a couple of audio books. I brought along some music CDs, my computer, and lots of snacks for my seventeen-year-old. I kept my husband Doug and daughter Beth, my son Caleb and his wife Hope—back home—current on our daily progress with a cyberspace travelogue on Facebook:

May 29, 2010:
AAA Triptik says our trip will take 3991.8 miles: First, to South Bend to see Andrew, then, to Grove City College to see the Munson family, to Gettysburg to see the Battlefield, to Virginia Beach for Peter to debate in national tournament, to Hardeeville to see our friends the Joyners, and finally, to Orlando to meet Doug for the Southern Baptist Convention. Peter and I have CDs, snacks, a GPS (Grampa's), maps, books — we are ready to go! (But of course we will also be taking Facebook.)

Chapter One

May 30, 2010:

Today ancient gospel singer George Beverly Shea on "Joshua Fit De Battle of Jericho," (etc), Loreena McKennit on "The Highwayman," or some such Celtic ballad, and Focus on the Family's "Silas Marner," together with lots of Cheetos, a couple sandwiches, and a long discussion on the sermon and some family history – gained Peter and me Blytheville, Arkansas.

May 31, 2010:

Today, Miles Gone By, *autobiography of William F. Buckley, narrated by the author, "Simple Gifts," "Glorious Things of Thee are Spoken," a couple of Bach pieces on Christopher Parkening's classical guitar, and a vigorous heartland rainstorm ushered us to Andrew's front door. He had chicken and rice waiting for us.*

June 2, 2010:

The dark recesses of the bachelors' lair have been scrubbed, shaken out, fluffed, and aired . . . in short, a slow transmogrification into a home that is cozy is taking place.

June 3, 2010:

Today: hospitality with Peter and Andrew – guests invited to a revitalized domestic atmosphere and served rosemaried salmon, baked potatoes, crisp asparagus, and corn on the cob, then ice cream for dessert. Compliments to Peter, the chef, while Mom and Andrew were running errands for the finishing touches on Andrew's house refurbishing.

Then, June 4, 2010, my entry of our day of earned recreation at Lake Michigan after a productive week:

Now I know where JMW Turner got his colors — sharp, true blues and greens. Chicago rose on the distant shore in blue haze. Beside me on a blade of grass crawled a ladybug with a gold sheen to her, tiny cubes of sand spread across her back. Kids played beside us. A boy did one handspring after another down the dune beside me. Another boy: "Lady, (to me) did you see how fast I rolled?" Peter and Andrew took turns snatching the frisbee off the air — beauty God gave us all richly to enjoy.

June 5, 2010:
Sigh. This morning we leave South Bend with hearts full of longing for more fellowship with our gentleman scholar. At least we leave him gleaming porcelain, two weeks of meals in the freezer, and every article of clothing he owns washed and put away. Now he can focus fully on studying for "comps," comprehensive exams to be taken on August 9. Pray for him, y'all.

The June 4 entry is emblazoned in my mind. We had packed a picnic lunch and travelled about an hour to Indiana Dunes National Lakeshore on Lake Michigan. None of us had ever seen the Great Lakes before. The startling blues and greens mesmerized and contented me for hours. I enjoyed my two sons quietly from my quilt in the sand. Though the sun shone warmly enough to lull me to drowsiness, the briskness of the wind leaping off the white crests of Lake Michigan kept me awake.

Behind the youthful grin, I could see the pastoral glint in Peter's eyes as he and Andrew plowed through the sand — it was not wet and packed enough to support their weight. Andrew huffed and puffed through soft sand to overtake the frisbee that kept playfully skipping on the wind just above his head, a gust in turn whisking it just beyond his reach. He had to jump hard from

Chapter One

a run to catch it. We saw his arms and legs stretching out to let go of the tension that his stressful semester had caused to accumulate in him. I saw Peter taking satisfaction; Andrew smiled.

As he watched the good he was doing to his older brother slowly take effect, Peter settled in for a frisbee marathon. I could read the thoughts that only revealed themselves by the twinkling lights in his eyes and a raised eyebrow: "I am going to skim this piece of plastic to that brother of mine till he drops." I am sure he must have wondered with me how long it had been since Andrew had exercised this vigorously.

They played frisbee throughout the afternoon. We had a picnic in the sand. Then we all three hiked the dune paths and the swampy Limberlost-looking woods beyond the lake. These two boys of mine are both nature lovers: in the early evening light, we spotted woodpeckers and finches and red-winged blackbirds and a whole mess of birds we couldn't identify. We clambered over a rickety wooden bridge, climbed a platform to an observation deck outfitted with public binoculars, and ended up hot, sweaty, and deliciously worn out. It was a perfect day.

This would be the last time the brothers would be together before their roles were reversed. Andrew would miss those exams he had been preparing for all summer. Two months later he would fly home to Peter's bedside, there to serve and show Pete the same gentle pastoral concern that his little brother had shown him — a vigil that would last long hours each day for months upon months.

Chapter Two

Thus began our longest journey together. — Harper Lee

It was Thursday morning, and Doug and I had just worked out together at the fitness center on seminary campus and had headed back home to start our day. Working out together had become our middle-aged date of choice, a productive outing that we both enjoyed. Though it hadn't done much for either of our figures, it provided some good stamina for ministry.

Peter had spent the night with his cousin; Nathan had coupons to Texas de Brazil, and the two had planned this last fling before Peter went off to college. They had stuffed their teenaged stomachs with meat. Peter was still gone when Doug and I had left to work out early that morning. While we were away, he had come home to change, greeted his sister, and then taken off in our old '93 Buick to drive the route we had driven hundreds of times, down the two-lane roads to our little church in the outlying community of Crowley south of Fort Worth.

He was off to mow and weed for Miss Alyce, our church's ninety-year-old heroine, a spunky widow who lived near the church. Declining health had only recently forced Miss Alyce to

Chapter Two

give up her yard work, to cease chucking rocks out of her garden and digging in hot Texas soil. She and her grandson had hired Peter to take up her work—Peter's friendly offering to relieve her of the heaviest tasks, and her contribution to Peter's college cash fund. (He would soon start at Union University, where he'd earned a partial academic scholarship to major in journalism.) Though Peter's great love was writing about history, he wasn't sure a historian could make a living if he didn't have a more marketable skill, such as those he would learn as he pursued Union's communications degree. He'd also earned a small speech and debate scholarship, so was eager to develop his parliamentary debate skills on Union's young debate team. Working for Miss Alyce was a way he could make up the shortfall in his financial package.

By 11:00 a.m., Doug had already put in a short morning of pastoring from his office at church, and I was on the phone trying to work out a last-minute vacation that we would take with our other children before I took off with Peter to settle him in at Union. With Caleb married and Andrew in Indiana, finding an open date that all of us could make had proved a challenge. We had finally nailed down a date in mid-August, when Andrew would finish comps and come down for a quick turnaround visit before the fall semester started up. As I talked on the phone to reserve rooms at a bed and breakfast cottage in South Texas, an unknown number beeped in. I ignored it. Whoever it was then called me on my cell phone. When I didn't answer it, Doug's cell phone, left behind that morning, jumped into action. *Someone is really trying to get a hold of us*, I thought. *Guess I better check it out.*

The woman on the other line was young, I could tell, but very calm. She identified herself as a nurse at the trauma hospital. She informed me that my son Peter had been involved in an accident about two hours previous and that I needed to come to the hospital right away. I asked her if it was serious. She didn't reply except to say I should probably come down quickly. She gave me directions to the hospital. I looked out the living room window and remembered I was without a car that morning. My daughter Beth was at the seminary, Doug had taken his car to church after our workout, and Peter had taken my car to work at Miss Alyce's house. I called Doug to tell him the news, in my muddled state thinking that I must wait for him to come home before I could make it to the hospital.

When I told him, Doug gave a loud, anguished cry. I encouraged him that maybe it had not been such a bad accident. Could he come home so that we could go to the hospital together? What I didn't know then was that it had immediately dawned on Doug that the wrecked car he had seen on his way to work that morning was actually our car, so twisted and mutilated that he had not recognized it then. As he had passed it, he had prayed, "O Lord, whoever was in that car, though it looks like no one could have lived through that horrible wreck, please be with them and spare them." It had shaken him. Now he realized in an awful agony that he had been praying for his own son.

It dawned on me that Beth was much closer to home than Doug was, so I called her to bring her car home, and then I jumped in the shower. I could go on to be with Peter, and she could wait for her father with the directions the nurse had given me. They could meet me at the hospital shortly. She sped home, a four-mile journey that still seemed to take too long. I headed out.

With all the effort it was taking to get us all coordinated to get to the hospital, I began to lose my calm. "Oh, my baby, my son!

Chapter Two

Lord, please help us here! Lord, my baby, my son, Peter!" was pretty much all I could pray as I sped to the hospital.

The reality I discovered at the hospital did nothing to diminish my prayers. As I learned of Peter's condition, I passed the information to those still not present. Beth and my daughter-in-law, Hope, immediately posted the news to Facebook, urging family and friends to begin praying for Pete's precious life:

On Facebook:

July 29, 2010: First Update
As many of you know, today at approximately 9 a.m. Peter Helms was in a serious car accident on Highway 1187. So far all we know is that he was t-boned by a Dodge pickup at around 60 mph. Currently he is in ICU at a hospital downtown and is suffering from severe head trauma after being taken there by helicopter. The surgeons were able to drill a hole in his skull this afternoon to release some of the pressure from the bleeding on his brain. As far as we know he has no severe injuries to the spinal cord or below his neck. However his condition is still very serious. He has several puncture wounds on his face and broken facial bones in addition to the bleeding on his brain. Please be in prayer for him and for the family. We will keep you updated as we can through this group. Thank you to those of you who have been praying or stopped by to visit today; it has been a great encouragement.

Within hours (thanks to Facebook), our friends and family all over Fort Worth and beyond had begun praying for Peter. Notes and messages like the one at the end of this chapter came flooding in. The first day in ICU, some three hundred Christian brothers and sisters showed up at the hospital to cry, pray, and wait with us.

On Facebook:

July 30, 2010
Today there has been no significant change in Peter's condition. The pressure from the bleeding on his brain has increased significantly overnight and the staff is doing its best to keep that under control through the tube the doctors inserted into Peter's head yesterday. Peter's pupils have only been minimally responsive to light. At this point, it is hard to tell if it is mostly due to the sedation he is under or his injuries. The neurosurgeon has encouraged us not to assume too much brain damage yet. Peter has injuries on the right side of his head near the temple, so the damage could be in the optical nerves. It will be several days before we have any more conclusive information.

On Monday or Tuesday, the doctors plan to try and get him conscious; but for now, they are just trying to keep Peter stable through this critical time.

Prayers for physical strength would be greatly appreciated. We are all exhausted (especially Mom, who was here through the night and has gotten very little sleep). God has used so many people to encourage and strengthen us, and we are so grateful.

We are sorrowful, yet hopeful, because we know we serve a God who can make even dead men walk again. God has been faithful to us in the past, even in our unfaithfulness to him, and we know he will be faithful to us as we walk the road ahead.

Thank you for your prayers!

"Where shall I go from your Spirit? Or where shall I flee from your presence? If I ascend to heaven, you are there! If I make my bed in Sheol, you are there! If I take the wings of the morning and dwell in the uttermost parts of the sea, even there your hand shall lead me, and your right hand shall hold me. If I say, 'Surely the darkness shall cover me, and the light about me be night,' even the darkness is not dark to you; the night is bright as the day, for darkness is as light with you." Psalm 139: 7-12

For the family,
Hope

The first night that Peter lived through the accident, I stayed with him. Somehow we had gained favor with the ICU staff, who had witnessed a barrage of fellowshipping Christians milling in and around their waiting room, many of them traversing the long corridor down to the last room where Peter lay. They patiently watched countless friends come and go, praying, hugging, weeping at his window. Eventually, when people arrived at the hospital information desk, they would say, "You are probably here for Peter Helms. He's third floor, corner room."

As we settled in for the night, I somehow drifted into a deep sleep. I awoke around 2:00 or 3:00 in the morning to a crowd of seven or eight medical people hovering around Peter's bed. They were shocking his heart. Somehow the crisis escaped my sleep-fogged brain, perhaps mercifully so. "Is everything okay?" I rose and asked. "Yes, he's stabilized now," someone answered. I turned over on the futon chair and fell asleep again.

The next day, another couple hundred people showed up at the hospital, supporting us, waiting, waiting. Doug and I began to take turns with Peter, one of us ever at his bedside, the other occasionally walking down to the waiting room to receive the love and concern that awaited us there.

On Facebook:

July 30, 2010
They ran an EKG (brain activity scan) and found that there are currently no seizures, and that Peter's brain activity is not flat-lined, so there is movement. As far as we know, he is doing as well as can be expected. Right now, it is critical we pray that Peter get no infections. He has so many ports and tubes, in addition to the head wounds, that this could happen very easily.

Also, tomorrow is mom's fiftieth birthday. God blessed us with a time of good family fellowship in celebration of her life last weekend and we are grateful for the memories. However, if you are coming by the hospital tomorrow, I know that she would really appreciate a card or other forms of encouragement.

Please continue to pray! I will keep you updated as I can and as new things occur.

Hope

Chapter Two

One of the things that I will ever be grateful for, considering all that happened later, is the fact that we celebrated my birthday a week early that year—five days before Pete's accident. Susan, my best friend from college, and her husband Blaine, brought over chicken enchiladas. Another pastor friend and his wife brought chips and salsa. The wife had been Andrew and Beth's violin teacher, and, since she and her husband had entered the ministry, they had become fast friends to our family. Caleb and Hope also arrived when Caleb got off work. Beth and I had cleaned the house earlier, while Peter finished off some work for Miss Alyce, arriving home in time to get a quick shower just before the others sat down at the table.

We Skyped Andrew in that night, perching the computer from which he looked out at us on the edge of the dining table, so that he could partake of the evening conversation. Though some of us were dubious that it would really work, we all gamely pitched in to speak clearly through the general din so that Andrew could join in. He had bought a frozen Mexican dinner to approximate what we were eating in Fort Worth. Hope, his new sister-in-law, kept a diligent watch on the volume and angle of the computer, doing her best to help Andrew hear and see and feel included in our evening's activities. It all had a rather comic aspect, but, of course, I was insistent that my oldest son be there for my fiftieth birthday celebration. Fellowship with my immediate family and close friends was all that I desired.

After supper, we gathered in the living room, and Doug led out in the yearly affirmation that we do for each family member on his birthday. I'll never forget our interchange that night. Andrew was saying that, though he'd had a hard year at Notre Dame, and was sometimes grumpy when we talked by phone, I'd maintained a cheerful demeanor and always sought to encourage him. "Thanks,

Mom," he said, "I really appreciate your consistent Christian encouragement to me, which you seem to be able to maintain even when I am melancholy."

"That's right, Selah," Susan echoed, a wondering lilt to her voice. "You are never grumpy."

At once, from the floor in front of the fireplace, Beth and Peter exchanged glances, Beth's eyes popping out, her mouth forming a dramatic "O," and Peter's expression not changing at all—only the characteristic twinkle in his eye and one quietly inclined brow. Apparently, they both thought Mom had another side to her that perhaps had escaped Susan and Andrew. I laughed, but pretended not to notice.

That raised eyebrow, so familiar to those of us who know Peter, was one of the first responses that he gave us to show us he was "there," weeks later, as he began his painfully slow ascent back to consciousness.

Late that night, after we had cleaned up the kitchen, Peter wrote a new Facebook status. A lover of family friendship as much as his mom, he revealed his pleasure in the evening. "Thank God," he wrote, "for the small foretastes of Heaven that he provides, like a restful evening enjoying the edifying fellowship of family and friends."

On Facebook:

July 31, 2010: Update
Peter is mostly the same today; he has made it through the first forty-eight hours! After the CT scan last night, the bleeding in his brain has gone down and we are cautiously hopeful. However, the doctors have told us

that we really need to pray the pressure in his brain will go down significantly. He has had a low-grade fever since yesterday, but has no infection. The staff says that he is pretty much where they expected him to be at this point. The nurses have been able to give Peter nutrition today through a tube, which they were unable to do yesterday because he had hiccups and they were concerned his body might try to throw up the nutrition. The nutrition should help build his immune system. The doctors have also told us that most of the time, when they see patients like Peter survive, only about 20 percent have full recovery, and 80 percent are severely disabled. We are still praising God that Peter has had no injuries to his vital organs or spinal cord as well as no broken bones besides the face. We know that God has been protecting him in many small yet significant ways.

Last night most of us were blessed with good sleep. Dad spent the night at the hospital and was able to get eight hours of sleep.

Yesterday we learned that someone joined the prayer group that was working nearby the scene of the accident and witnessed everything. We learned that this person was able to go to Peter and comfort him, which may have saved Pete's life. We have been so grateful to hear this news and it has comforted us.

Thank you again for all of the support you have been giving us. Here is a message from mom:

"All of you, thank you so much for the prayers. We feel carried along by the prayers of God's people and by the grace and love of the Lord. We have heard that there are people praying for our boy in the United States, Mexico, England, Germany, Peru, Korea, Kazakhstan, China, France,

Slovakia, Mali, the Amazon, and the Philippines. He is in the Lord's gentle hands. Please keep praying. The next couple of days are critical."

For the family,
Hope

Those first few days, we heard from all over the country. Friends I hadn't talked to in ages called me on my cell phone. From my vigil beside Peter's bed, I was rarely able to take the calls immediately, so I listened in the evenings to each day's accumulated messages. Each woman who called spoke my name in the tenderest way as she began her message. I knew each one felt the desperation in my mother's heart.

By Sunday, we were hearing from all over the world, a product, I guess, of my pastor husband's genial way of forming strong friendships in missions and ministry over the years, multiplied by the quick spread of information the computer afforded to a very connected Christian community. One long-time pastor's wife friend from California told us that on Sunday morning they'd arrived at church, ready to give Peter's name to their church family and enlist their prayer support. "Oh, we already know about Peter and are praying for him," one woman said.

My daughter Beth, a sophomore at the College at Southwestern Seminary, was contacted by a classmate, who had flown home to his native Hawaii for the summer. On the Wednesday night following Pete's accident, this young man had traveled out to a remote congregation off the back roads in Hawaii to minister. When he arrived, the church was praying. A woman asked for prayer for a Texas homeschool family named the Helms whose son had been in a bad car accident. He immediately recognized that this must be Beth's younger brother, and he wrote to encourage her with news of these far-flung prayers.

By Sunday night, we had heard from Christians from over thirty countries who were praying for Peter. These people were telling us that they were up in the middle of the night praying for Peter, that God had laid him on their hearts intensely, and that they couldn't stop praying for him. One of my best friends related how her daughter, Heidi, a friend of Peter's in our homeschool co-op, had come into her room that night, deeply disturbed. Both she and her mom felt that Peter might be about to die. They got down on their knees and begged God for his life. We figured that with the time differences around the globe, Peter was being prayed for around the clock. We received many notes like the one below.

Hi Doug and Selah,
You all have been on my mind and heart. I couldn't help but think of you all and the trial you're going through. I have prayed for you several times a day. What I wrote below has come to mind, and though it doesn't seem near as good typed up as in my mind, I hope that it will encourage you just from considering that there is much more going on here than we can see.

"Now there was a day when the sons of God came to present themselves before the LORD, and Satan also came among them. And the LORD said to Satan, 'From where do you come?' So Satan answered the LORD and said, 'From going to and fro on the earth, and from walking back and forth on it.' Then the LORD said to Satan, 'Have you considered my servant Doug, that there is none like him on the earth, a blameless and upright

man, one who believes in the sovereignty of God and the sufficiency of scripture?' So Satan answered the LORD and said, 'Does Doug fear God for nothing? Have you not made a hedge around him, around his household, and around all that he has on every side? You have blessed him with a Proverbs 31 wife, sons and a daughter that fear you, a daughter-in-law that fits right in the Helms family, and a church that takes the Bible seriously. But now, stretch out your hand and touch one that he has, and he will surely curse you to your face!' And the LORD said to Satan, 'Behold, the one he has is in your power; only do not take his life.' So Satan went out from the presence of the LORD.

"Now there was a day when his son was on his way to a widow's house when an unseen pickup truck slammed into his car. He was careflighted to the hospital with an unknown future. In all this, Doug did not sin or charge God with wrong."

"For our light affliction, which is but for a moment, is working for us a far more exceeding and eternal weight of glory, while we do not look at the things which are seen, but at the things which are not seen. For the things which are seen are temporary, but the things which are not seen are eternal." 2 Corinthians 4:17, 18

"For I consider that the sufferings of this present time are not worthy to be compared with the glory which shall be revealed in us." Romans 8:18

We love and appreciate you all and wish we could see you more often.
David

Chapter Three

Whether I live to see you a man, or not, I hope you will work in the Lord's vineyard wherever he calls. I never asked anything for you but usefulness, in all my prayers for you, never once.
—Elizabeth Prentiss (spoken mother to son)

From the time Peter first asked about spiritual things, he had a humble honesty. He lacked the self-consciousness that keeps some children shy about making themselves vulnerable to their parents. He opened his heart freely to his dad and me. His questions revealed that he truly understood the struggle for supremacy going on in his own heart.

We had set out years earlier to rear our children in the love of the Lord. We wanted to give them a vision that all of life was a vehicle to love God more, whether learning or serving, working or playing. All of life's experiences merely afforded more opportunities to know Jesus Christ better and to make him better known. We wanted to walk through life with our children, giving them a vision for this at every turn.

Beth "caught" this one day when we were planting flowers in our front garden: "Mommy!" she exclaimed, "We're planting flowers, and the flowers are really beautiful, and that glorifies God!"

"Yes," I answered. "True."

"And we are working, and work glorifies God," she chattered eagerly on. "And we are doing our work cheerfully and our cheerfulness glorifies God too!"

This was the vision we wanted each of them to catch. They cut their teeth on the children's Baptist version of the Westminster catechism—What is the chief end of man? To glorify God and enjoy him forever—and as they grew older, the diligent study of beauty and goodness and truth showed up in the way we approached history, literature, and the arts as we enjoyed what we learned of the Lord there.

It was simple, really: we just wanted them to worship God in all things. This spiritual simplicity made its way into many of Peter's journal entries from his childhood. True, many of the pages are filled with stories he created that read like *Lord of the Rings* epics with different character names, or detective stories that sported the protagonist "Sherlock *Helms*" —his own childish renditions of himself solving all kinds of adventurous mysteries. He also wrote extensively on the paintball wars in which he and his brothers fought. But it's when he wrote of his daily life, that his young spirit shines through. Peter wrote the entries below the year he turned nine. He remembers the time we learned of the plight of the Sudanese people, many of whom were being captured and sold as slaves. Our kids, troubled by the realization of suffering outside their comfortable lives, persuaded their cousins to earn money with them raking autumn leaves—enough to free a Christian slave, valued at one hundred dollars at the time. Our children, ages seven,

Chapter Three

nine, eleven, and thirteen, plus their four cousins of roughly the same ages, earned enough for two "purchases." I have left Peter's childish impressions and misspellings intact:

August 3, 2001

Today is Friday. We are going to Six Flags, that is, if we get our school done. I know I am going to be a ckoward like I was the other times, but I hope and think I will have a very good time. I have been to Six Flags two times. Both times I was a ckoward. But I hope all of us have a good time and glorify the Lord. . . . Some minutes later: I CAN GO TO SIX FLAGS – all school work is done!!!

August 6, 2001

Today is Monday. I want to write about us maybe freeing a slave out of slavery, either with our family and/or with the children of our church. About a year ago, we freed two slaves by raking leafs for people with our cosins. We have a cheerful giver jar. Everybody should give what they think they should give. The cheerful giver jar has 11 dollars and a slave costs 100 dollars. So we are still a long way away. I hope we do free some slaves if it's God's will.

August 13, 2001

Today is Monday. I want to write about . . . my birthday! It was on Saturday. It was a very fun day and yesterday we got to go to the Roberts house. From Grace I got a notebook and from Joel I got tictacs and from Holly a beany and from Anna and Emily I got gum. When we were at our own house, Joe spent the night and gave me paintball gloves and a beany. From Gramma and Grampa Weaver I got a paintball gun and from the other grandparents $25 and mom and dad gave me a paintball mask and Beth gave me Legos and from Caleb I got paintballs and from Andrew I got a tether ball thing and from some of our friends I got a car and pencils. So you see even thow I had a little birthday, I had a fun time. I hope I glorified the Lord too.

Memories of these early birthday celebrations passed through my mind in those first few days of the hospital stay following Peter's accident. I wrote entries for the website as I sat by Peter's side through those long hours, waiting, watching, hoping. Remembering vestiges of his childhood prayers, I couldn't help but be comforted. Peter's youthful convictions trickled into the self-talk with which I comforted myself as I contemplated his chances of surviving this ordeal, especially since my fiftieth birthday arrived two days after his accident, "celebrated" while he was in ICU:

On Facebook:

July 31, 2010: Message from Peter's Mom
Thank you so much, all of you, for your concern and prayers. Those prayers for my son are the best birthday gift anyone could give me today, on my fiftieth birthday.

I've thought a lot today about our family birthdays. And I'd like to share with you something about Peter that comes to my mind (since many of you do not know him).

For many years, Peter's dad has led each birthday celebration by having a time of affirmation and blessing for that particular family member. After each of us in turn had encouraged the birthday celebrant, we would pray together.

Chapter Three

The Lord gave Peter a grateful spirit from an early age. Beginning around age seven, during the prayer following his affirmation time, Peter would pray, "Lord, thank you for these seven good years you have given me. And Lord, if you are so good as to give me another year, I want to use it to glorify you." Then off to bed he'd go, perhaps holding one of his new toys.

Then on his eighth birthday, the same: "Lord, you've been so good to give me these eight good years. You have given me so much more than I deserve. Lord, if you are so kind as to give me another year, help me to glorify you with it."

Every year he remembered to do this. No one coached him in it. And as he grew, we could see the fruit of the Lord's work in his life.

So today I want to follow my son's example: My prayer request on this birthday is that God would be glorified. If the Lord so chooses to make this a part of my life message and my husband's and that of my other children, we want to make the most of the opportunity to praise his beautiful name. We trust God to do whatever he will. But I'm asking as well, that the Lord will make this a part of Peter's own life message, that the Lord will raise him up and restore him to glorify the Lord by his own mouth once again.

The Lord is worthy of anything he asks us to walk through for his purposes. I want to use it to show how good he is.

"How sweet a thing were it for us to learn to make our burdens light by framing our hearts to the burden, and making our Lord's will a law."

— From The Loveliness of Christ *by Samuel Rutherford.*

August 1, 2010: Update
Nothing has really changed this evening. I think there are just three main prayer concerns right now:

1. *That the pressure from the bleeding on Peter's brain would be dramatically reduced. This evening it has been pretty high, and higher than most of the day.*
2. *That he would not throw up any of the nutrition he is getting through a tube while he is on the ventilator. If he were to get the nutrition in his lungs he could develop pneumonia, which we want to avoid. The nutrition is important to help his body heal itself.*
3. *That the swelling in all areas of his body would be reduced as much as possible.*

We are thankful for each and every one of you who is praying on Peter's behalf!

August 2, 2010

Today the staff took Peter off the sedatives in order to see if he can breathe on his own. He has been unresponsive, but we are not sure how much of that is due to the significant quantity of sedatives he has been given over the last three days. Peter was unable to breathe on his own, so it looks like they will be doing a tracheotomy to help his breathing long-term.

This morning his left pupil was slightly more responsive to light than it has been and the intracranial pressure (ICP) went down very slightly. Continue to pray these will improve, and also pray that he will eventually be able to breathe on his own and wake up from the coma at the right time.

Chapter Three

Thank you again for all of your prayers and support. We have been overwhelmed by God's provision for us during this time and we have always had plenty of food here at the hospital to cover our needs. We also wanted to thank those of you who have shared stories of God's faithfulness in similar situations in your lives. It has provided great encouragement.

Hope

August 3, 2010: Evening Update
Peter is still in very critical condition, but we see very small signs of possible improvement that encourage us greatly. This evening we have read Scripture to him and talked to him a little bit. Right now the pressure in his brain is doing well enough that they are not giving him any sedatives. This increases the chances he can eventually breathe on his own or wake up from the coma.

Earlier today Peter did not have much physical response to our touch, but tonight sometimes the left side of his body will move a slight amount. Right now there is no way to tell whether or not this is a reflexive or cognitive response, but it is such a delight each time it happens. We miss being able to interact with Peter.

Continue to pray for the following things:
1. *That the pressure/swelling in his brain will continue to decline and will stay down. His ICP numbers have been pretty steadily below twenty today (which is what they want to keep it under) compared to the last couple of days where they got in the middle-to-high thirties. This is a praise, but keep praying in this regard.*
2. *Continue to pray against infection. It is always a risk, but Peter seems to be doing well so far.*

3. Pray that in the next few days when the respiratory therapist does a series of tests on Peter's breathing, that Peter will gradually be able to breathe on his own. Right now they are waiting to do a tracheotomy until Wednesday, so there is plenty of time for improvement in his breathing before then.
4. Continue to pray for the physical health of our family as we try to be here for Peter. Pray for good rest, and that we would be free of sickness so we can be at Peter's bedside as much as possible. Pray for spiritual and emotional strength as well during our long hours here at the hospital.

Please bear with me as I write these updates. It is difficult to get the facts straight because every report varies depending on the nurse or doctor and sometimes the reports get a little muddy in our minds. I will continue to send out the best information I have as frequently as I can!

"When the righteous cry for help, the Lord hears and delivers them out of all their troubles. The Lord is near to the brokenhearted and saves the crushed in spirit. Many are the afflictions of the righteous but the Lord delivers him out of them all. He keeps all his bones; not one of them is broken. The Lord redeems the life of his servants; none of those who take refuge in him will be condemned." Psalm 34:17-20; 22

For the family,
Hope

The constant yearning of our broken hearts, hour after hour, for a sign of life and consciousness in Peter, was interspersed with countless visits from friends and well-wishers wanting to help in some

Chapter Three

way. Even the hospital staff showed unusual care for Peter. Couriers from our governor arrived with a hand-signed book for Peter, who had completed his Eagle Scout project the night before his accident. The book on Eagle Scouting was written by Governor Perry—he had heard about Peter and wanted him to know he was praying for him. Prayer groups showed up, wanting to pray over Peter, some to anoint him with oil. One man told us he belonged to a "high-end prayer group" that was guaranteed to get results. His daughter walked down the ICU hallway with me to Peter's room. She told me that Peter's example had inspired her to live for the Lord as she contemplated going off to college. Hearts went out to the young man who showed such promise, so ready to be useful in life and so suddenly cut down. Below are some of the messages we received in those early days, a legible demonstration of the Lord's care for us, prompting his people to be his hands, his feet, and his voice.

Dear Doug, Selah, Andrew, Caleb, Hope, Beth... I wake up early with my husband and I'm addicted to the "Pray for Peter" site. It's amazing but not surprising to see how our Lord is using you and especially Peter through all of this. Your gentle, powerful, faithful service as a family has been a challenge to me personally over the years. . . . I was hoping you were talking directly to Peter, knowing that he most likely hears and senses your presence. . . . I was wondering if there is a nurse family member or friend available with you to explain basic things (IV infiltrating and hand swelling etc, wish I was there with you). Hope has done an awesome job weeding through all of the info you get from the medical staff and conveying it to all of us waiting to hear the next piece of news.
Carol Geraldo

Get used to seeing me . . . daily . . . lots of love. Get well li'l dude.
Steve Godley

Precious Helms family...I have to tell you that we are praying daily and often for Peter in our household. My husband is one of the ICU nurses (he introduced himself to you all last week). I have to say that your family is a HUGE testimony to God's amazing grace, sovereignty and mercy to a huge staff of doctors and nurses up there. There are many people who are watching how you handle this difficult providence and you are having an incredible opportunity to shine the truth of the gospel before an unbelieving audience in a way that you would never have otherwise chosen. God IS being glorified in this situation through the faith and hope you all are expressing. What an incredible encouragement you have been to me as I've read this page and seen the way you have expressed trust in our mighty God. We will continue to constantly lift Peter and all of you before God's throne of grace to find your help in this time of need!
Kelly Lester

I LOVE your comments for today, Peter's mom . . . witnessing to others through this, I mean offering a call to salvation not just having them watch what you are dealing with and seeing how God is moving, is VERY moving to me! Thank you for sharing this!
Teresa Johnson

Peter and your family have always been an incredible inspiration and source of encouragement to me in my walk with God. I pray for Peter's healing and that God would send comfort and peace to all of you. God is being glorified through this. "How deep the Father's love for us, how vast beyond all measure, that he should give his only Son, to make a wretch his treasure."
Timothy Wilson

Chapter Three

I don't know Peter, but my friend asked me to pray, and I joined your group. God works in mysterious ways. I have read the daily updates on Peter and messages from the family. You just don't know how inspiring and how it has blessed my heart to read these messages. I know that the main objective is for Peter to be healed, but you know, the Lord may be using Peter to inspire others. God bless you all, and please heal Peter!
Terry McCartney

My sweet four-year-old Anna is constantly asking to look at pictures of Peter and after we looked at some this morning, she said, "We need to pray for Peter all the time because we miss him and he's our friend." Then she asked that we pray for him right now and she prayed for him. We do all miss you and love you, Peter, and are praying constantly for you!!
Heather James

I just received an invitation to pray for this young man and his family. It is my absolute honor to do so. I know you know that the Lord is sovereign in all things. He is also merciful!! I will be praying for complete healing. What a witness that will be!! Love in the Lord,
Cathy Hilton

Hello, you don't know me but we have the same Father. I want to encourage you with the reminder that he is there with you in that hospital, as you wait on the Doctor's next report, as you watch Peter. . . He cares so much for you. I am praying that you rest in his love and presence today. He's got Peter, and you all, in his loving Hands. Grace and Peace to you.
Joy Perrey

From Colombia my family is praying for Peter's recovery! God Bless! Mrs. Helms, you don't know me, I met your father last month in Colombia

on a mission trip...He let me know what's happening. Even though, we trust in a God who gives us MIRACLES every day. Count on our prayers, Peter will GET WELL!
Stephen Martel

In your last communication, August 2, you said that there were over 1900 praying. There are probably many more. I am one of those who have been praying, but who has not communicated with you. And I am, no doubt, one of many. Thank you for allowing us to be a part of God's ministry to you during this time. Continuing in prayer,
Shirley Davidson

Greetings from Cowboys For Christ International. Brother Don DeFoor sent me a message the night of Peter's accident requesting we start a "prayer chain." We sent a message to over 2300 members around the world. Prayers and replies began to pour in immediately, streaming in well into the night and beginning again the next morning. We have very many anointed intercessory prayer warriors who interceded for Peter and have been praying for the family. We love Peter and the Helms family and are believing God for a miracle and total, complete healing, in Jesus' Name. Let us know if we can be a blessing to you in any way.
Doris Bailey on behalf of CFC International (Our headquarters are here in Fort Worth)

Hi, I don't know Peter, I just saw this on a friend's page and was drawn to it. I've read all of the updates available, and you all are in my thoughts and prayers. May the Lord keep Peter in his hands and heart, as well as keep all of you strong. Your faith has been an inspiration to work on strengthening my own. God Bless you,
Cathy Blanchard

Chapter Three

Hey Peter,

I just want you to know that I'm praying for you. You know John Piper's book "Don't Waste Your Life". . . well, from what I've heard and read about you, it sounds like you were living that — using your life to make much of our King! Your witness has been a challenge to me. And I know that you must be glad to have a family who lives this as well, a family who hasn't wasted your accident! Keep going strong, brother . . . and remember that God is using this to make you and your family more like Jesus. . . . His wounds were deep as well!

Your brother in Christ,
Matthew White

Only four days out from the accident, over 1900 people were praying for Peter and following his progress. Many of them had never even met our son. We were grateful and humbled.

As we sent out updates to our allies, I tried to acquaint them a little more with the young man for whom they prayed.

Peter's senior year had been very uneven: we had planned a family wedding as parents of the groom, cared for a godly Gramma before she went to be with the Lord, and borne some ministry heartaches. These things had put heavy demands on our time. In all this, Peter had quietly picked up on the needs of others and pitched in to help serve, counsel, and bear their burdens. He was calming in stressful situations.

One day, I told him, "Son, I apologize for how crazy your senior year has been. I feel like I haven't given you or your schooling nearly enough attention. I have neglected you."

Peter, an easy-going, unassuming guy, always answered with a ready smile. "That's okay, Mom," he told me. "I know you love me. I'm just grateful to be a part of your and Dad's ministry."

That thought comforted us at his bedside. While he was an eager student and a quick learner, Pete's heart had long been moved to serve the Lord. He would be pleased to know that he was serving as a catalyst to draw the Body of Christ together and inspire Christian service.

We would sometimes read through Peter's Bible aloud as we took turns sitting at his bedside. One verse he highlighted: "The Lord is a stronghold for the oppressed, a stronghold in times of trouble. And those who know your name put their trust in you, for you, O Lord, have not forsaken those who seek you." Psalm 9:9, 10

On Facebook:

August 4, 2010: Update
Nothing has changed today. No new response or movements different from yesterday. The doctors have said they will probably try to remove the stint in Peter's brain because the longer it is in there the higher the risk of infection. At this point the pressure is under enough control that an infection would be worse than more pressure on his brain.

Right now we are trying to shift towards a more long-term mindset since Peter is in his own coma. I am not sure how much this has hit us yet, but we have not lost confidence in our God. We continue to read Scripture to Peter and talk to him and let him know he is never alone.

We appreciate your prayers so much. As we feel so loved through your prayers, we realize even more that our hope is not in the number of prayers ascending up to heaven on Peter's behalf but in our mighty God who hears those prayers. We know God may not choose to heal Pete, but we also know he is capable of restoring Pete to full health and we will not cease to pray for that.

For the family,
Hope

August 5, 2010
Today the doctor's plan is to remove the stint in Peter's brain and adjust the sensor that is measuring the ICP. The sensor went out a couple of days ago and they have been unable to get accurate readings since then. The outside of Peter's face looks a lot better today. He also has a fairly high fever, but other than that, there are no changes to his condition. Our family was able to get some good rest last night, which is a definite praise.

Here are the main prayer concerns for today:
1. *That as the doctors perform the procedure for the stint, everything will go smoothly, and also that God would protect Peter from infection in that area. Doing the procedure increases the risk of infection.*
2. *Continue to pray against pneumonia. From what I understand the risk of pneumonia is pretty high when you have a machine breathing for you, but more so on the ventilator versus the trach. Since Peter has not been given a tracheotomy yet, this is still a big concern.*
The family has also asked that for those of you who would like to come visit, please come before 8:30 p.m. in order for Peter and

> *the family to get more rest. We appreciate that you come to see us, so feel free to come during the day.*
>
> *We are grateful for all of you!*

We had no doubt at the time that Peter would want us to use his accident as a platform to shout the good news of Jesus Christ and his gripping love for those who trust him. We shared the gospel freely in those days. And in the face of the possible death of our beloved son, no one could dispute the strength of such a message. I don't know if any became believers, but everyone was willing to listen to people who could deliver such a message at such a time. When we could weave in Peter's experience, it seemed to pack a punch that the same truths spoken outside of suffering lacked.

On Facebook:

August 6, 2010: Message from Mom
Today I'd like to share with you the blessed hope we have at this difficult time. The Helms family stands united in declaring to you that we have no strength or merit of our own with which to meet life's demands or sorrows. Our hope is in the Lord, who gave himself for us.

Peter would tell you freely, if he could right now, that he falls short of any goodness of his own, and as his mom, I would add that he has his various assortment of teenage hangups, several that we have been challenging him on before he heads off to college.

Chapter Three

Prior to encounters with Christ, we believe that, as sinners, we were all in the act of running away from God, and as his enemies, were unable to see beyond our own shallow desires and selfishness. When we wanted something so bad that we were willing to sin to get it, we revealed idols in our own hearts that we worshiped more than the Lord. Thankfully, the Lord opened Peter's eyes several years ago to see the beauty of Jesus Christ and his sacrificial love for us. What an amazing thing that, "For our sake he made him to be sin, who knew no sin, so that in him we might become the righteousness of God!" (2 Corinthians 5:21) Jesus bore God's anger for the very sins we committed in chasing after other things more than him.

When Peter was a child, there was a time when we were memorizing 1 John 2:15, 16: "Do not love the world or anything in the world. If anyone loves the world, the love of the Father is not in him. . . ." Peter came to me later, troubled, and confessed, "Mom, I don't think I'm a Christian because there are things in the world that I love more than God." Peter's Dad and I discussed this with him over the course of several months. We took him to Matthew 22:37: "You shall love the Lord your God with all *your heart and with* all *your soul, and with* all *your mind." He began asking God to change his heart, to give him a love for the Lord, and to save him from his sins.*

At one point, he told us that he was sure he loved his parents more than God. I reminded him of Christmas and asked him, "Peter, when you receive a gift from Mom and Dad at Christmas, do you like the gift more, or Mom and Dad more?"

He answered, "That's easy. I love you and Dad more; why would I love the gift more?"

"Son," I said, "Look at it this way. The Lord is the giver of these things you love. Mom and Dad and these other things are only the gift. The giver of the gift shows the love – it's not the gift itself that shows it. God is the one you should love, because he is the one who is being kind to you."

Eventually the Lord opened Pete's eyes and brought him to the point of surrender. "Mom," he told me one night in earnest, childlike sobriety, "I am ready to give all I have to Jesus and even to give my life for him."

For our Lord Jesus is the pearl of great price, precious enough for us to yield all we are and have. With his parents, Peter has acutely realized the daily need to embrace a life of continual repentance from selfish desires, and, by grace, to treasure the Lord more and more.

"My hope is in the Lord who gave himself for me,
And paid the price for all my sins on Calvary.

"No merit of my own his anger to suppress,
My only hope is found in Jesus' righteousness.

"For me, he died; for me, he lives,
and everlasting light and life he freely gives."

Chapter Four

Everyone then who hears these words of mine and does them will be like a wise man who built his house on the rock. And the rain fell, and the floods came, and the winds blew and beat on that house, but it did not fall, because it had been founded on the rock. And everyone who hears these words of mine and does not do them will be like a foolish man who built his house on the sand. And the rain fell, and the floods came, and the winds blew and beat against that house, and it fell, and great was the fall of it. — Matthew 7:24-27

The chances we had to speak a word for Christ were laid out like a red carpet for us continually. We kept a family member with Peter twenty-four, seven in those early days. His life still hung in the balance so precariously. The hospital staff became accustomed to having us at their elbows. Several appreciated it when we took an interest and listened attentively to their explanations of what they were doing. One respiratory therapist, Jo, was on duty for several days in Pete's room. We chatted with her, talking freely of the Lord, as she gave him breathing treatments. She liked Peter and often spoke gently to him. Though friendly, Jo had a sharp edge to her. A nurse told us she struggled with sadness around this time every year because of a deep loss she had sustained in her own life.

One day, Jo told me she really wanted to talk to me. I said I could at once. She said, no, she wanted to wait until she was off duty. She asked me to talk to her the upcoming Saturday, when the hospital load would be lighter, after she got off work. I said I would.

When the day arrived, she sought me out, just coming in for my turn at Peter's bedside. We found a spot in the lobby that was quiet. We sat down, and I looked at her. Jo's eyes flashed bitter fire.

"I want to know," she demanded, "where was God when Peter had his accident?"

"Well," I replied, "we believe that God was there when Peter had his accident, and that even traffic accidents cannot separate us from the love of God."

"Well, it makes me angry," she said. "God could have prevented it and he didn't!"

Yes, I had to agree with that—he didn't. But why was *she* so indignant about it?

She teared up, drawing a small spiral notebook out of her scrub pocket. She located a certain page, and a worn photo of a beautiful young woman and a crinkly-smiled baby fell into her fingers.

"This was my daughter, my only child, and this was my granddaughter. In this picture, my daughter is thirty years old and my grandbaby would have turned one the next month."

By this time, sobs were overtaking her.

"They were both killed the same day in a car wreck. They were all I had. I lost everything, and I am so angry."

Chapter Four

It was a touching revelation. My heart, having recently sustained its own wound, bled easily with hers. She related what a good person her daughter had been—a churchgoer, a Sunday school teacher, a loving mother, and a devoted daughter. She didn't deserve to die.

"We are taught that God is in charge," she said. "Do you believe that?"

I said I did.

"Then why didn't he protect her that day? It's not fair! They were all I had!" she repeated.

I tried to explain that God is love as well as he is sovereign, and that he intends love towards us. Spoken from the bedside of Peter's suffering, I knew my words carried weight.

She told me that she had tried to be an atheist, but failed. "I knew I was angry. And if I was angry, it had to be directed at *someone*. So I knew I wasn't an atheist."

I asked her if she would be willing to read something, and she insisted she would not. As she grew more agitated, I decided to be more direct.

"Jo," I said, "You are thinking like an American."

"What do you mean?" she asked.

"I mean, you are acting as if you deserve things. You have an attitude of entitlement. You could try being grateful for what you had. How many people in this world were blessed, like you, to have a daughter that was lovely and a good person? Many people are not blessed with children at all. And those who have children don't always have children who turn out well. You had a daughter who brought joy to you and others for thirty years. You could try to be grateful for that. God has been good to you and given you more than you deserve. That's how I try to comfort myself about

Peter. He is only seventeen, but he has been a good son to me. And no matter what happens, I am trying to be grateful for the years we have had with him. You will lose the reality of God's goodness if you let yourself drown in a sense of entitlement."

She listened, said little in response. But I saw her again in Peter's room a few days later. She was tender towards him, then came and embraced me. "You were right about the sense of entitlement," she said.

As Peter's hospital stay stretched longer, Doug, our children, and I began to help with Peter's care. One day, as Doug was at Peter's bedside helping change his sheets and hospital gown, the nurse began to criticize men. "Yeah," she said to me, "your husband and Andrew are an exception to the rule. Most men you couldn't even keep in a hospital room for more than five minutes, much less see them actually helping. Men don't like to do hard things—too irresponsible!" We knew that she was a single mother working hard to make ends meet.

"Well," I replied, "that's the difference Christ makes in a man's life. It makes him want to take responsibility and to care for a family. Christ changes a man's value system." She looked dubious, but what could she say in the face of the daily gallantry she saw in my graying, fifty-ish husband?

Every day we spent in the hospital I saw the fruit of Doug's diligence to build his family on the foundation of Scripture. I thought back to our first year of married life, the year we memorized the book of Ephesians together. How my gratitude swelled for Doug, who loved God's Word so much from the time of his youth. When our children arrived, he began reading aloud to them each night, for thirty or forty-five minutes at a time when they got old enough. While he read, we let them draw or color, which kept their eager hands busy and did not seem to hinder their ability to listen to their dad's voice in Scripture. And we made allowances for the occasional trip to the bathroom, or to the kitchen for a drink. They could even come and go from mom's lap for a little cuddling, as long as they were quiet. Doug would ask them questions after he closed the Bible, and to our delight, we saw that having their hands busy not only kept their voices quiet, but seemed to increase their powers of comprehension as well.

By the time Peter's accident struck our lives, Doug had read through the Bible in his personal devotions each year for the past several years, sometimes the New Testament through twice in a year. This practice had seasoned his speech with wisdom and his mid-life with stability and gentleness. We had made it through many vicissitudes of ministry, largely due to the bedrock of Bible grounding his heart. And as God had used past trials to establish this bedrock, our family and our marriage had grown sturdy. But little had I known before how much I would now come to rely on my husband's spiritual strength.

Every father and husband has his weaknesses, and every family its "issues" to work through, but children will seldom rebel against a father figure they see as ready to admit his own weaknesses and guided by a trusted authority higher than him. Our kids knew that Doug wanted their spiritual success for their own sakes. Peter spent his early years on his stomach, drawing pictures and absorbing holy words that he realized were important, as Doug read. His early journal entries are shaped by the scriptural thoughts expressed by his faithful dad. And his own copy of the Word, when he became of age to glean on his own, was marked throughout with his own interactive reflections on Scripture. We would soon discover that nothing but a foundation laid on the Word would hold firm in the storm of suffering we and our son would face.

Here again are entries from his journal at age nine:

August 22, 2001

Prayer is talking to God. If we use prayer the right way, God will be pleased. Some times when we ask for something, he says "yes" but sometimes "no." This is how I sometimes pray, "Dear Lord, please help me to glorify You" and "please use me." "I don't deserve to have any good thing you give me." "Please forgive me of my sins." "Your will be done. In Jesus' name, Amen." That is how I sometimes pray.

August 23, 2001
What is a Godly man like?

A godly man does not have to be the Apostle Paul or some of the twelve, but godly men glorify God and godly men do what God wants them to do. I know a lot of godly men and one is my dad because he preaches God's word. Grampa is a godly man because he gives. My other grampa is a godly man because he is very encoriging and helps me. And when I grow up I want to be a very godly man.

August 25, 2001
My favorite artist is Rembrandt. He is my favorite artist because he makes it look very normal. He used his family and friends for models and thought of his father as a very wealthy man. In one of his works of his mother, her hand looks so real; it looks like you could touch it. Rembrandt liked dogs and put them in some of his pictures. Rembrandt drew some Bible pictures and was probably a Christian. That is who my favorite artist is.

Chapter Four

September 2, 2001
A good friend is someone that loves at all times. A good friend is someone that shares and considers others interests before their own. A good friend is someone who encourages you when you need it. A good friend is someone that you learn from and they learn from you. Mom and Dad are good friends to me. Andrew, Caleb and Beth are good friends to me. I have a lot of good friends, but surely there is no greater friend than Jesus. That is what a good friend is like.

September 3, 2001
Today is Monday. I want to write about Joshua. We have not known him very long, but we are already becoming friends with him. Oh yes, we have not told you where he came from. He is Mrs. Rosemary Duncan's foster child. We have had him over to spend the night with us. Yesterday we had him over for lunch and watched a movie and then played outside. It was a very fun time and I hope and think that we glorified the Lord.

Nine years skimmed by. Our children became adults, and the Lord began to answer Peter's childhood desire to glorify himself.

On Facebook:

August 7, 2010: Message from Dad
Our hearts are filled with gratitude to the Lord for how kind he has been to us in all of the last week's trauma. He is a great God and a Sovereign Lord. I love the prayer of Nebuchadnezzar recorded in Daniel 4:35, ". . . He does according to his will among the host of heaven and among the inhabitants of the earth; and none can stay his hand or say to him, 'What have you done?'" The God we serve is sovereign: there is no one above

him telling him how he should govern his world. And none of us can harness his power to serve our own purposes. He uses his power to do his will and to bring glory to his name.

And yet, at the same time, he is a kind and loving God, a Father to those who come to him by faith in his Son Jesus. He has dealt with the Helms family as a loving and gentle Father. His promise to his own is that he will never leave us or forsake us. As Romans tells us, "For I am sure that neither death nor life, nor angels or rulers, nor things present nor things to come, nor powers, nor height, nor depth, nor anything else in all creation will be able to separate us from the love of God in Christ Jesus our Lord."

So our greatest comfort in this calamity has been that our son Peter is in Christ, and even during this serious wreck, he was never for a moment separated from the love of God. And we ourselves have felt his presence and love throughout this week.

At the same time, we are praying fervently with all of you for Peter's healing. We know the Lord hears our prayers. Yesterday we met for the first time with a doctor from the next floor, where Peter will go from ICU. We talked about therapy and rehabilitation. This is to us wonderful news in light of where we were a week ago.

We have been speaking to Peter, reading Scripture, singing hymns to him, and reminding him of who he is and who we are in relation to him, in hopes of making his transition back to us easier. We've been told we should play some of his favorite music to him. Since Peter is a pianist, his grandfather suggested that we play music for him that he performed in the last couple of years — since he would be so familiar with it. His cousins have begun to put some music on his iPod.

Chapter Four

Each year, our church family holds a summer Scripture memory contest for toddlers through seniors. One year Peter memorized the entire book of James and quoted it to his church family. We have found places in his Bible where he targeted certain chapters for memorization. Peter was faithful to hide God's Word in his heart. So we are putting the book of James and other passages he's memorized on his iPod as well. Our prayer is that God will use some of the good habits that Peter developed to help bring him back mentally, spiritually, emotionally, and physically.

Please continue to pray that his fever will drop and for grace and wisdom for the next phase of recovery. Our God is amazing. Thank you for your prayers. We love you.

Doug

August 8, 2010: Saturday Update
Late last night the doctors performed the tracheotomy and feeding tube procedures and they went very well. Peter looks much more comfortable with the trach.

Peter has been off sedation since 7 a.m. and has had a very quiet day. We are not too worried that he hasn't woken up yet since he was under general anesthesia for the surgery. It's not uncommon to have a day with slower progress after a few exciting days.

Here are the main prayers concerns right now:

1. *Peter's fever. Peter is on an antibiotic for the pneumonia but his fever is still 103. The nurses are getting cultures done to try to localize the problem so they can treat it effectively.*

2. Peter is in his own coma, so be in prayer that his brain/head will be restored and that he will wake up and be able to regain full use of his brain.

Thank you all!

For the family,
Hope

August 9, 2010: Message from Mom
In Peter's NKJV Bible, this Sunday morning, as I sit in his hospital room, I found the following verses underlined in the book of Isaiah (with Peter's comments in brackets beside each verse, parenthetical comments mine): change divine pronouns from version's practice?

"'For a mere moment I have forsaken you, but with great mercies I will gather you. With a little wrath I hid My face from you for a moment; but with everlasting kindness I will have mercy on you,' says the LORD, your Redeemer." — Isaiah 54:7, 8 [This is the basis for perseverance.]

"Why do you spend money for what is not bread, and your wages for what does not satisfy? Listen carefully to Me, and eat what is good, and let your soul delight itself in abundance." — Isaiah 55:2, 3 [A Christian seeks greater pleasure than the world. The world's problems are that it seeks after too little pleasure — that which does not satisfy. God is the greatest pleasure.]

"All your children shall be taught by the Lord, and great shall be the peace of your children." — Isaiah 54:12 [Is this me? Pray for peace and joy in the Lord.]

Chapter Four

"The work of righteousness will be peace. And the effect of righteousness, quietness and assurance forever." — Isaiah 32:17 [Not happiness, but the things that make happiness.]

"The Lord is exalted, for He dwells on high, He has filled Zion with justice and righteousness. Wisdom and knowledge will be the stability of your times, and the strength of salvation. The fear of the Lord is his treasure." — Isaiah 33:5, 6 [Good verses to meditate on.]

"Your eyes will see the King in His beauty; they will see the land that is very far off." — Isaiah 33:17 [The Sands of Time — Emmanuel's land (a reference to one of Peter's favorite hymns), Delectable Mountains (I think a reference to Pilgrim's Progress).]

" . . . and [Hezekiah] said, 'Remember now, O Lord, I pray, how I have walked before You in truth and with a loyal heart, and have done what is good in Your sight.' And Hezekiah wept bitterly." — Isaiah 38:3 [Depending on our own goodness doesn't give us peace or rest.]

"O Lord, I am oppressed; Undertake for me! What shall I say? He has both spoken to me, and He Himself has done it. . . . Indeed it was for my own peace that I had great bitterness; but You have lovingly delivered my soul from the pit of corruption, for You have cast all my sins behind Your back." — Isaiah 38:14, 15, 17 [Pleading the Lord to undertake for us gives peace and joy.]

"So Hezekiah said to Isaiah, 'The word of the Lord which you have spoken is good!' For he said, 'At least there will be peace and truth in my days.'" — Isaiah 39:8 [Where is the multigenerational faithfulness thing?

(reference to his exposure to Voddie Baucham's ministry) Meditate Isaiah 40 — strong chapter.]

"'You are My witnesses,' says the Lord, 'and My servant whom I have chosen, that you may know and believe Me, and understand that I am He. Before Me there was no God formed, nor shall there be after Me. I, even I, am the Lord, and besides Me there is no Savior.'" — Isaiah 43:10 *[If you want to know what the Lord thinks of Himself, read Isaiah . . . and tell others. Against Jehovah's Witnesses: Jesus is called Savior.]*

"Put me in remembrance; Let us contend together; state your case, that you may be acquitted." — Isaiah 43:26 *["Till We Have Faces" (Peter likes this book by C.S. Lewis.)]*

Every Sunday morning that Pete spent in the hospital those first few weeks after his accident, we spent with him reading to him from his own Bible — a practice that ministered to us as much as we hoped it did to Pete. On several occasions, I posted other listings of verses accompanied by Peter's comments like those above. We have included these subsequent entries in Appendix A at the end of the book.

August 10, 2010
It has been about three days since Peter's tracheotomy and he is still pretty deep in his own coma, just making minor movements and probably nothing intentional (although time will tell). The doctors have given him a medicine today that is supposed to help stimulate brain activity. They

Chapter Four

are being pretty aggressive about trying to wake him up. As far as I know, there have still been no major changes since he has received the medicine to help wake him up. We are just trying to be patient.

Pete's fever has gone down some, but they still haven't located the source of the infection. The respiratory therapist has also been slowly weaning Peter off of the ventilator, and his own breathing seems to be improving!

Another question to be faced is what to do after Peter can breathe on his own if he hasn't woken up from the coma. Rehab facilities won't take him until he is awake, tracking, and following simple commands. He will probably move to another floor in the hospital for a while between ICU and rehab, but no definite plans have been made.

Here are the things to pray for:
1. *The pneumonia/infection Peter has. It would be a wonderful blessing for these to go away.*
2. *Continue to pray for Peter's full recovery and the restoration of his brain functions.*
3. *Pray that Peter's breathing will continue to improve.*

Depending on how much progress Peter makes in a day, these updates could be spread out a bit farther. If that happens, please continue to pray over the things in the previous update and anything else the Lord lays on your heart.

For the family,
Hope

Chapter Five

The most extraordinary thing in the world is an ordinary man and his ordinary wife and their ordinary children. —G.K. Chesterton

Part of what made Peter's accident so poignant to me was the fact that he was an intelligent high school graduate, on his way to a scholarshipped college career and eager to be useful to God, when he was cut down. He was only seventeen. We would celebrate his eighteenth birthday in ICU with a very different affirmation time than the one with which we'd planned to send him off to Union University two weeks later. He had been packed and ready to go.

When our friends at Union received word of Peter's accident, a multitude (it seemed) promptly joined in the prayer vigil for his survival. We heard that David Dockery, the president of the university, had asked the Union community to pray for Peter during the summer commencement ceremony. One of the admissions people from the school showed up later to visit us at the hospital. A recruiter called with a message from Dr. Dockery that when Peter recovered, there would be a full scholarship waiting for him at Union. Further, if he needed family assistance at that time, his sister Beth, currently in college, would be welcome to accompany him, and she too would be granted a full scholarship. It was a magnanimous gesture.

Of course, we had no idea whether he would ever go to college at this point, but I inwardly rejoiced that Peter's heart had always gripped learning intensely. I knew that my son had learned to worship through his studies, and that he had pursued the knowledge of God through his curiosity. In our study, we didn't merely gather trivial facts; we constructed a framework of thought that helped us understand our own life histories.

So years ago, when our children wonderingly watched the jets hurtle into the Twin Towers, we asked what perspective history can give us to understand what was happening. Had evil been allowed to succeed like this before? What had good people done about it? We read the story of the ten Boom family, and how they chose to face the evil in their generation.

And when my mom's cancer recurred after eleven years of remission, we had a great cloud of witnesses whose life stories we were familiar with, to give us insight into her needs as well as to help us encourage her in her suffering. This was what our "school" was for.

When, in 2006, a tornado smashed into the campus of Union University, where Peter's older brother Caleb was a resident assistant, but not a student was killed, we immediately recognized it as an instance of God's providence that has been so plentiful in the lives of his saints throughout history. We had read enough about Christians in history to recognize the providence of God in things that seemed to turn out right . . . or wrong. Peter's childhood journal (age nine) discloses his youthful understanding of these heavy issues.

September 5, 2001
Today is Wednesday. I want to write about school starting up. I am glad about it in some ways and not in others. Some of the reasons why I'm glad is because we're doing spelling. I'm also meeting with Dad. We're doing co-op school and devotion. Some of the reasons why I don't like it is because of grammar. But I hope I do it with a cheerful heart. I also hope we have a good time and glorify the Lord.

September 11, 2001
Today is Tuesday. I want to write about a catastrofy that happened today in New York City and Washington, D.C. Thousands of people died. How it happened is that a plane crashed on purpose and it was by a terrorist group from Palastine. They are going to probably try to fite every body on Isreal's side and we are some of those people. We watched the news and it was a tragedy. I hope the familys that their loved ones died would be encouraged but most of all them to become Christians by this tragic catastrofy.

September 12, 2001
Today is Wednesday. I want to write about me being content about my family. I am very content about being in this family. God put all of us in the right family and we need to be gratefuller for our families. Some parents are too harsh or too un-harsh. But wether they're harsh or not harsh, the best you can have is a Christian home. But some children don't even have a mom or dad. So I encourage you to be grateful for any mom or dad or brother or sister, and remember that God put you in that family for a very good purpose.

Chapter Five

September 26, 2001

Today is Wednesday. I want to write about the Chaselys and Roberts who came over early today. It was very fun. They came over to do co-op school and later we played outside. Holly and I had a very suiting lunch in a tree. In co-op school we were studying about early American history and for our project we started a Jamestown motel. While Holly and I worked on the gate around Jamestown, Beth and Anna did the houses. We did not finnish it today, but we got a good start on it. Some of the stuff was for strong hands, and some of it was for careful hands but we came out of the mess soon. But it was a good craft time, and I hope we glorified the Lord in everything.

October 4, 2001

Today is Thursday. I am going to write about Holly, Isaac and I being in a Bible Study group with each other every Wednesday. We decided Wednesday night, and Wednesday morning I was unhappy because I thought that I did not have any boys with which to do a Bible Study group. But I was overjoyed when Isaac said he would do it with Holly and me. Holly was not prepared, so we only had prayer requests, prayed, and looked up things in the Bible and took notes. But it was very profitable, and I hope we did and do learn from each other, and not just do it to check it off the list, but do it to become better Christians.

On Facebook:

August 11, 2010: Message from the hospital; The Train Ticket
I saw a post on the PRAY FOR PETER HELMS group page that sparked my interest (one of many that do), and I decided to comment. It was

*Chasity McClure's post about the train ticket story from the life of Corrie ten Boom (*The Hiding Place*).*

Many of you are familiar with the story from ten Boom's childhood when, going to minister to a woman whose baby had died, she was first confronted with the reality of death. She became terrified that one of her own loved ones might die, certain she could never bear such a thing. Seeing her distress, her father wisely instructed her that the Lord gives us the strength to bear things as they come to us, and not before. Just as he himself had dealt with her as a father at the train station, giving her her ticket only just prior to boarding the train, the Lord gives grace to bear what we will be called upon to bear just before we need it.

I assure you moms out there that I have battled all the things any mother's heart would in a crisis like this: grief, fear, anxiety, fatigue, discouragement. Three weeks ago, I don't know that I could have born the events of this past week and a half. But let me share with you the thoughts that tumbled through my mind as I raced to the hospital last Thursday. (I hit every light on red and ended up behind the slowest drivers in Fort Worth. It was maddening.)

Days earlier, I had reread a couple of books that I commend to you. The first was Tim Ellsworth's book God in the Whirlwind, *the story of the tornado that wrecked the campus of Union University in February 2006. If you read that book, it will truly lead you to worship as you see how the Lord directed every piece of flying debris and every room that exploded in such a way as to spare each student's life, even those who didn't take the warnings seriously and who were not taking appropriate cover. One student was saved by a gumball machine that prevented a concrete wall from crushing him. Another was saved when a sofa flew across the room, pinned him to the ground, and sheltered him from a falling wall. The Lord's hand covered each of these students with personal, divine attention, so that, though responders initially expected scores of fatalities, not a one was lost.*

The other book I reread was an old favorite of mine, the semi-autobiographical novel Stepping Heavenward *by Elizabeth Prentiss. Prentiss was a dear godly woman who has mentored me over the years as I have been rereading her books since I was thirteen. The following passage, written from a mother's perspective, tells how her family faced a serious illness in a young daughter:*

One morning she seemed almost gone, and we knelt around her with bursting hearts, to commend her parting soul to him in whose arms we were about to place her. But it seemed as if all he asked of us was to come to that point, for then he gave her back to us, and she is still ours, only sevenfold dearer. I was so thankful to see dear Ernest's faith triumphing over his heart, and making him so ready to give up even this little lamb without a word. Yes, we will give our children to him if he asks for them. He shall never have to snatch them from us by force.

The thoughts from this remarkable and rich incidence of God's Providence (my son Caleb lived through the tornado as a Union student), coupled with the yielded meekness portrayed by Mrs. Prentiss, fortified my heart with fresh truth twelve days ago. If the Lord asked for my son, I wanted to yield to him, knowing that his hand would never cease to spare or save when it served his holy will.

Selah

As mentioned above, on the evening of Peter's eighteenth birthday we had a time of family celebration around his bedside. We all took turns touching Pete and telling him what we appreciated about him. Then we ended in a good time of prayer and singing.

That evening Peter was moved out of ICU to another floor. This meant that he was stable enough to no longer need the intensive care that ICU provided.

Peter had resumed breathing on his own during the day, but needed the ventilator's assistance at night to save his strength. With his fever finally coming down, and his pneumonia clearing up, we were so grateful.

We began doing some physical therapy with Pete and establishing a routine of reading to him and letting him hear things he had memorized to help stimulate brain activity.

Still, Peter showed little response, especially compared to the week previous. Sometimes his eyes would be partially open, but they stared blankly and we could see that he wasn't conscious.

On Facebook:

August 12, 2010: Birthday Poem for Peter
Written by Rosemary for Peter's eighteenth birthday, the day we moved him from ICU:
A Birthday Surrender in honor of Peter on his eighteenth birthday

August 11, 2010
Every life, no matter how idle,
is marked with a beginning day;

it's part of God's common grace to man —
he gives him life, even if he seeks his own way.

But for the man who seeks his own way,
though grace is there, it is less
than the abundant grace that a man of surrender
receives when he makes "gaining Christ" his success.

For the man who pursues his Savior
and can say in his heart, "to die is gain,"
is a man who has been set apart by God
to serve him, in joy or in pain.

I know such a man who has been set apart,
a child of God from his youth,
who willingly served his Master
and sought to live by truth.

Even if it meant working hard
to love God more than anything else:
his toys, his "collection," and even his parents —
he was determined to not live for self.

And, by God's grace, he learned what it meant
to surrender his affections to the Lord.
He knew that whatever the cost of the call
was a price his soul could afford.

He knew such a life meant surrenders,
and selfish pleasures he couldn't pursue,

but loved his God more than those things
and said, "What he asks, I will do."

And each year, as he grew one year older
the refrain of his prayer rang true:
"You've given me more than I deserve.
If you give me more life, let me live it for you."

And today, as he grows another year older,
he would say the same prayer if he could,
so until he can, we'll say it for him,
and trust in the Lord, who is good

to answer this prayer as he wills,
for that is what Peter would say —
"If you are so good as to give me more life…"
and then trust God for each new day.

So, Lord, we trust you this day,
and echo Peter's birthday prayer.
We want his life to glorify you,
and we surrender him into your care.

We lay our affections at your feet;
we lay Peter there too.
And say, as his heart learned to say from his youth,
"What you ask, we will do."

For you are worthy of everything,
of all we have to give.

Chapter Five

*We join with Peter to say from our hearts,
we will serve you as long as we live!
Happy Birthday, Peter!*

Things were relatively quiet with Peter, and we were gradually moving into a routine. To wean him off the ventilator, the respiratory therapists challenged Pete to breathe on his own in the mornings and daytime, then they put him back on the ventilator at night to help him rest. His independent breathing improved, but slowly.

Though Peter's responsiveness was still minimal, there were small daily flickers to encourage us. At the same time, he was having spells of agitation, when his heart rate would spike and his breathing would become labored. We didn't know whether these problems and his fever were due to pain or to his injured brain's inability to regulate those things.

We prayed that if Peter was in pain, he would be treated with just enough narcotic to ease the pain, but not too much to keep him from waking up.

On Facebook:

August 18, 2010: Update
Yesterday Peter was really relaxed in his coma. The previous days since he was moved out of ICU seemed more agitating and traumatic for him, so it was nice to see. He just looked peaceful.

He still has quite a bit of fluid in his lungs and sometimes coughs so hard we see tears come from the corners of his eyes. It's hard to watch. Pete's fever continues to go up and down throughout the day. We think that the fever issues are partially due to his inability to control his body temperature due to the head trauma.

Responsiveness is still minimal.

Chapter Six

When we read the poem, or see the play or picture or hear the music, it is as though a light were turned on us. We say: "Ah! I recognize that! That is something which I obscurely felt to be going on in and about me, but I didn't know what it was and couldn't express it. But now the artist has . . . imaged it forth . . . for me, I can possess and take hold of it and make it my own, and turn it into a source of knowledge and strength." — Dorothy Sayers

When Peter was around six, we put him in a small, local art class. The teacher told the students to draw pictures of their favorite toys. Peter promptly drew a pencil and an eraser as carefully and accurately as he could. From his journal:

September 6, 2001
Today is Thursday. I want to write about one of my hobbies. My number one play thing I like to do is drawing. You may not call that playing, but it is to me. I draw every day. It is very fun and I think I'm okay at it. I do think I like to draw the most in our family. And this is hard to believe, but I started at two. I love to draw more than any playing thing and I hope I glorify the Lord with my drawings.

As he grew up in our homeschool setting, I tried to give Peter lots of opportunity to exercise this propensity to express his life in pencil. Even into high school, we used a multi-media approach to learning that gave artistic bent a lot of room for expression. In our small, home-based Western Civilization class of about ten students, we trekked through Ancient Greece and Rome, the Middle Ages, Renaissance and Reformation, and into Modern Times with all kinds of hands-on projects to facilitate the students' delight in the great books.

Andrew gave us the ultimate compliment when he arrived home from college the year of Ancient Rome (for our high schoolers). He proclaimed that our little homeschool production of *Julius Caesar* topped anything he had seen produced by the University Shakespeare team.

When we studied Dante's *Inferno*, a sibling set in our class crafted a Lego staircase, each step illustrating one of Dante's nine circles of hell, their little Lego men stirring pots of punishment with little plastic smiles on their faces. Peter drew a large poster board depiction of the nine circles of punishment, Virgil in his toga and Dante in his Italian finery hovering above the scene in colored pencil.

During our medieval study, one student delivered a presentation accompanied by a visual aid—an arrow stuck through a play-doh eye, which showed why Britain had lost the Battle of Hastings to William the Conqueror in 1066 (King Harold was shot that way). The student, dressed up as "Matilda," the dwarf wife of William, presented to the class the Bayeux Tapestry, Matilda's work, still extant, which narrated the story on fabric.

For a final project, the class collaborated on a ten-minute *tour de force* through the Middle Ages and Reformation—complete with recitations from the Magna Charta, King Alfred's Doom book, the Koran, and Luther's Ninety-five Theses. Each student appeared and reappeared in multiple historical roles. Peter played a feudal vassal, the prophet Mohammed, Henry V, Martin Luther, and a marauding Gaul. Beth figured as Joan of Arc, an Augustinian monk, a crusader, and a baron of King John Lackland. Other class members represented the Dauphin of France, Pope Urban II, Augustine of Kent, and other important history shapers. Some students compiled a complex soundtrack: Gregorian chants for the monastic scenes, trumpet blasts for heraldic proclamations, a thundering voice from heaven to bestow Mohammed's vision, and Lord of the Rings music to underscore the many clashing wooden sword fights that the boys eagerly scripted into the play.

We brought allusions to Peter's classical Christian education into his hospital room in hopes of stimulating memories for him as he recovered consciousness:

On Facebook:

August 20, 2010: Waiting…in the Hospital
Today marks the beginning of the fourth week since Peter's car accident. The doctors and nurses tell us that, though it seems like a long wait to us, it's actually still very early on in the recovery process for an injury like Pete's.

My husband reminds me often (and I'm thankful) that we are not just waiting on Peter to wake up, but that we are also learning to wait on the Lord, and that there are promises in Scripture for those who wait on him. I really like C.J. Mahaney's definition of waiting on the Lord. It showed up in a post by Sunny Fraser on the group wall: "It takes faith to wait tranquilly for something for which we have a promise from God, but no date. . . . Waiting is not resignation; waiting is active trust in God to provide fulfillment in his perfect timing, according to his ultimate purpose of glorifying his Son."

As we wait on the Lord "more than the watchmen wait for the morning," he promises to renew our strength. He also promises that he will give what is good to his children, just as an earthly father would – that if we ask him for bread, he won't give us a stone. So we come to him fully trusting his character, asking for bread. Then, we wait. But we know while we wait that in whatever manner God chooses to give to us, what he gives will be bread and not a stone. We cry out to the Lord, asking for many things regarding Peter's healing, and we know his answer will be good and will come in his perfect timing.

People ask me how I'm doing. Well, as I'm learning to wait, here's what I am doing: the duty of this particular day. It's a discipline included in waiting – that I learn what my duty is only for the day at hand, without giving in to speculating on future days.

What is trust and what is obedience for this day? I'll tell you what it looks like, practically speaking. For one thing, I am learning much about physical therapy and respiratory therapy. We do Passive Range of Motion (PROM) exercises with Peter throughout the day, and talk to him about things he is familiar with. Here's the schedule we have been loosely adhering to around the interruptions that typically happen in hospital life:

Chapter Six

7:00 a.m. — Family member who spent the night with Peter wakes up. Miriam (dear friend who was once an ER nurse, now homeschooling mom of Peter's good friend Caleb) arrives. She goes through PROM with Peter, talks about date, time, and weather, sings "Give Thanks" to him, and reads Isaiah 40. Nurses come through and give him meds.

9:00 a.m. — PROM with Dad. Doug reads through questions #1-5 of the Shorter Catechism with Peter, including scriptural proofs. (Peter memorized the Shorter Catechism in high school.) Doug sings "Before the Throne of God Above," prays with Peter, and talks to him. He also reads James 1, as Peter memorized this in the past.

11:00 a.m. — PROM with Doug again, then questions #6-10 of Shorter Catechism. Doug then sings another hymn, reads James 2, and talks to Pete. Then we put on YoYo Ma playing the Unaccompanied Bach Cello Suites in the background. It's soothing.

2:00 p.m. — PROM with Selah. Then I read James 3 to Peter, talk to him, and sing "Great is Thy Faithfulness." Often I also read Shakespeare's version of King Henry's Saint Crispin's Day speech before the battle of Agincourt. As an avid history buff, Pete chose this as another piece of memory work a couple of years ago.

4:00 p.m. — PROM with Selah again. Then James 4 and "Great is Thy Faithfulness" again. Then I either put on "Eine Kleine Nachtmusik" and some other Mozart, or some of the pieces Peter has recently performed in piano recitals.

7:00 p.m. — PROM with Andrew. Then Andrew reads James 5 to him, and we all sing "Jesus, I My Cross Have Taken" around his bed. This is *often the song Pete chooses for his turn during family devotions. When Caleb, Hope, and Beth are there, it really sounds good because they sing in parts. We miss Pete, though, because Peter's the only one in the family who sings the bass line, so it doesn't sound as fully rounded without him. We hope he can hear the difference, and that it will prompt him to wake up and help us out.*

Last night, Andrew and I were trying to be creative in coming up with new things to talk to Peter about. "Twenty Questions" has been an old family favorite from the time the kids were young. So we played it over Pete's bed. Andrew guessed Knight Roland and Neville Chamberlain from my clues. I guessed Bede, but got stumped on King Hrothgar. So Andrew won. Pete would have guessed King Hrothgar.

"Wait for the Lord; be strong, and let your heart take courage; wait for the Lord!" Psalm 27:14

Selah

August 23, 2010: Sunday Update
Peter has been making slow but steady progress towards breathing entirely on his own. His fever has also been down today. As soon as Peter is ready, we plan on bringing him home to take care of him until he can go to rehab.

Peter still only shows slight movement and not really any direct response to commands. We are praying this will change as he comes closer to waking up.

This past week Peter's fever broke, but we think the recent fluctuations have him quite worn out. We are grateful that his brain functions are starting to work again to keep his body temperature more regulated.

For the family,
Hope

August 24, 2010: New Prayer Request
Last night Peter had a really difficult night. He coughed a lot and was unable to breathe on his own or do the breathing challenges. The nurses think that it might be a bug of some sort (like a respiratory infection). It has been a setback for him, and the nurses are getting cultures done to see if they can find the problem.

Please be praying that Peter can fight against infection and that God will protect him from it as well. The longer he stays in the hospital, the more he is at risk for the hospital bugs that are resistant to antibiotics. It would be horrible if he had to deal with that while he is healing and in the coma.

For the family,
Hope

You know, I have always been an earthbound girl. From the time I was young, I had wholehearted ambitions about what I wanted to accomplish in my life. My goal in raising my children was to gear them to make an impact on their world and claim ground for the kingdom of Christ. I had dreams of a child of mine going on the mission field, one into academia, one into law, and one into music, all claiming every square inch in their respective disciplines for the Lordship of Jesus Christ.

As I sat by Peter's hospital bed, I wrestled with confusion. Peter was so outfitted for usefulness and so eager to enter the fray on Christ's side. I couldn't understand why the Lord would sideline him. Peter was intelligent, yes, but more importantly, he was humble and sincere. Highly intelligent people who are proud can end up not being very useful, but Peter was so different. His humility seemed to make him a person that God could really bless as he found his place in the world. Doug and I were sure that in either a pastorate or a writing career, Peter would be careful and honest and diligent in all he contributed. Why did this not seem more important to God than Peter's current condition would indicate? It made no sense to my understanding of God's calling.

I began to believe that the Lord might actually be unclenching my fingers from their hold on the world and focusing my desires into an ambition for heaven. Maybe I hadn't valued heaven enough. Maybe I was selling my Christian life short by setting my sights too low. Perhaps Peter's life would not be as useful on earth as it would be in heaven. Or perhaps the Lord would have Peter give up his chance to make a contribution here on earth in order to help the rest of us prepare more scrupulously for heaven. Maybe the sacrifice of Peter's life was for my benefit; my son would help his mom, his dad, his siblings, and perhaps others outfit themselves for a much more important destination.

Strange as it sounds, the picture of Michelangelo's *Pieta* kept coming to my mind as I watched over Peter's limp body in the same sorrowful manner that Mary attended to her son. Of course, Peter was no Savior, but many dust-bound saints in history have given their lives for the Lord's higher purposes. Would Peter be one of them? Would God use Peter's suffering for some bigger plan of his own? And as I saw people that I only barely knew in our broader Christian community begin to make sacrifice after sacrifice in their time and treasure to help us in our crisis with Peter, I couldn't escape the thought that the Lord would like to see all his children willing to give their lives for each other. Isn't that what Christian community is all about?

On Facebook:

August 26, 2010: Peter's Art; A Message from Mom
Today my desire is to share a little more about Peter. I liked Craig Sivil's post yesterday that gave a brief glimpse into his life in the National Christian Forensics and Communications Association. Speech and Debate was a large part of Peter's life during his last two years of high school.

Peter is also a gifted artist. His very earliest characters were no mere stick figures. Even those first drawings held a lot of wit and insight. When he was seven, he entered the Fort Worth Stock Show Art Contest and took first place in his age division. He went on to place in following years as well.

Peter's cousins related the time Peter got in trouble in a classroom. A few kids were doodling on paper while a film was being shown. Peter was the only one called down for it. And the teacher threatened to tell his parents if he continued "doodling." Why? Because Peter's "doodling" was an elaborate scene of a knight on a raging battlefield of men and horses.

As a literary family (or as one of our friends has lovingly pointed out after reading these entries—as a family of "geeks"), we have read through many books over the years. Peter has always been fascinated with the literary idea of the "Christ figure"—a person in the story who lives beyond his years in kindness and understanding, or who ends up bearing the weight of another's struggle, who forgives another at great personal cost, or who sacrificially lays down his life for someone else in the story. Such characters function as a "type" of Christ in these stories.

Two of Peter's most beautiful pieces of art are from a series he began three or four years ago (but then became busy with high school and never finished) of Christ figures from stories we've read. After reading David Copperfield *by Charles Dickens, Peter fashioned a clay figure of the young Ham dashing into the waves towards a sinking passenger ship. (At peril to his own life, Ham ends up rescuing a young man who turns out to be the rake who steals his fianceé.)*

Another story Peter likes is Victor Hugo's Les Miserables, *so he sculpted an aging Jean Valjean bearing a wounded young man on his back through the gutters of Paris in order to rescue him from battle. This young Marius is suitor to Valjean's adopted daughter—the girl to whom Valjean is devoted and for whom he has sacrificed his whole life. Marius was the young man who would woo her away from him.*

Pete was planning another clay figure of Sidney Carton (from Dickens' A Tale of Two Cities) *on his way to the guillotine to die in the place of the gentlemanly husband of the woman Carton secretly loves. Peter had also considered sculpting Uncle Tom, the Christ figure from Harriet Beecher Stowe's Civil War era novel.*

Chapter Six

I don't want to glamorize Pete, but I do like to think that the suffering he's experiencing on his hospital bed is accomplishing spiritual work in us all. May the Lord make it so. I do know that your sacrificial prayers, love, and support (meals, cards, green juice, hosts for the waiting room lobby, contributions, visits, house cleanings, house preparations to make ready for Peter, lawn mowings, and so much more) have certainly undergirded us with God's grace.

"By this we know love, that he laid down his life for us, and we ought to lay down our lives for the brothers." 1 John 3:16

Selah

August 27, 2010: Update on Peter's infection

The doctors have been unable to localize the infection and Peter's white blood cell count is really high (which means his body is trying to fight whatever it is), even though he is on an antibiotic. They are taking cultures again, so please be praying that they can find the source of Peter's infection. Thank you.

For the family,
Hope

Throughout those high school years, some of Peter's closest friends were Zach, Heidi, and Nathan Hughes, all of them students in my five-year Western Civilization course. Heidi provided this tongue-in-cheek narrative of our goals as we made our way through the Great Books:

Zach looked upon my outburst indulgently, as he always did. He didn't seem to care that our carefree days of youth were being eaten up with toil. He didn't seem to realize that it was his cause as well as my own that I championed to Mom.

"Four o'clock. Till four o'clock! That's how long it takes us to finish homework every day. In our books we study Beauty, but don't get to see the sun's beautiful light until it is nearly set. I don't expect Mrs. Helms to relent, but you, my own mother, can hardly look on while we are driven so."

My melodramatic plea was met gently, but with no sign of liberation. I tried again.

"Beth told me that the tests take hours to finish. Beth's writing hand is cramped for days afterward. This isn't school; this is slavery."

Mom said that Mrs. Helms' history/literature class was a non-negotiable part of mine and Zach's schooling, and that one day I would appreciate it.

I didn't think I'd survive long enough to appreciate anything.

I knew, of course—we all did—why we did it. At the start of each new school year, Mrs. Helms would give students old and new her "Why We Study the Classics" lecture. Themes of loyalty, justice, and fallenness (and their many cousins); touchstones of goodness, truth, and beauty; the eternal cycle of tragedy and redemption—these were things that we and other students of the Classics were being trained to quest after in each new book, to trace in the ebb and flow of civilization, and eventually, to map out in our own corner of history. We must discover, by studying the

Chapter Six

original sources from a Christian standpoint, not just how things used to be, but why and to what purpose. We must apply these lessons to our own time and see how our world today came to be, and how we ought to respond. By the early Medieval period, it was starting to come together for me: that modern students inherit the humanism of the Renaissance, the emotionalism of the Romantics, the empiricism of the Enlightenment, the hubris of ancient Greeks and Shakespeare's Macbeth alike, and must therefore arm to fight anew many of the same battles our ancestors did; that the books they left to us hold the Excalibur of our age; that great men are usually counter-cultural (and often a bit eccentric); and that in the worst and darkest — Bubonic Plague or the fall of an empire — there is always a remnant of God's people.

We knew exactly why we agonized over dusty books and pondered the lives of skeletons now moldering in Westminster Abbey.

Every man's last day is fixed.
Lifetimes are brief, and not to be regained,
For all mankind. But by their deeds to make
Their fame last: that is labor for the brave.
Below the walls of Troy so many sons
Of gods went down… Turnus, too, is called by fate.
He stands at the given limit of his years.
Aeneid, 10.650-655

"Isn't it beautiful, Heidi?" Mrs. Helms would say. Of course it was, but I didn't want to admit it, especially to Mrs. Helms, whom I feared on principle. I loved to read, but until then, fun books and school books had been distinctly separate, and I thought it proper to keep them that way. To admit that a person could enjoy mandatory labor would be weakness.

> But Beowulf was mindful of his mighty strength,
> The wondrous gifts God had showered on him:
> He relied for help on the Lord of All,
> On his care and favour. So he overcame the foe,
> Brought down the hell-brute. Broken and bowed,
> Outcast from all sweetness, the enemy of mankind
> Made for his death-den.
> *Beowulf*, 1266-1276

"Isn't it beautiful, Heidi?"

"I guess so."

Fine. I liked learning. I liked thinking. Of course I liked good books. But to say so would be to admit a kind of defeat, wouldn't it?

> Once more into the breach, dear friends, once more,
> Or close the wall up with our English dead!
> … On, on, you noble English,
> Whose blood is fet from fathers of war-proof…
> And you, good yeomen,
> Whose limbs were made in England, show us here
> The mettle of your pasture. …The game's afoot.
> Follow your spirit, and upon this charge
> Cry "God for Harry, England, and Saint George!"
> *Henry V* 3.1.1-40

"Isn't it magnificent, Mrs. Helms?"

She knew I was conquered.

The heftiness of the material didn't mean we hadn't any fun. Mrs. Helms liked to punctuate long weeks of book-grind with a class project, or what she called "fun assignments." There were even games on a regular basis—the week before each test. Like a prisoner's last feast before the scaffold, it was a sober joy. Many of Mrs. Helms' fun assignments were designed with an eye toward rounding out our creative abilities. So, during our study of Merry Robin Hood, each of his twenty-first century admirers composed a ballad to be sung or recited in class after the tradition of Ye Olde Troubadour. Some sang scholarly riddles in iambic meter; others, oppressed by the task, chanted dolefully of underfed monks. But it was Peter's minstrelsy, a parody of Johnny Cash's "Man in Black," that carried the day. Pete sang of the Man in Green, whose daring exploits in Sherwood Forest were equaled only by his brightness of spirit and greenness of gear. Even our unassuming poet himself barely suppressed a grin at the last chanting of his refrain, "…that's why I always dress in green, why mine's a cheerful mien," massaging the pronunciations of "green" and "mien" to coax a rhyme.

Next term, Dante's Inferno, in its many-tiered grimness, was laid upon our artistic abilities. Beth brought a neat illustrated chart of sinners' eternal punishments, labeled in order of atrocity. My brother and I hauled a scaled model of Hell into the Helms' living room (our classroom, affectionately nicknamed "The Dungeon")—yellow Lego men toiling behind boulders, steaming in pitch, and waiting to ferry the River of Death with all the impenitence of printed plastic smiles. No one was surprised when Peter unveiled, with a dismissive chuckle, a colored-pencil masterpiece of Roman poet Virgil leading a dismayed Dante through a gauntlet of fire and demons.

Another time, it was a panel discussion, and students in the various guises and doctrines of Iain Murray, Billy Graham, Jonathan Edwards, and company argued the Great Awakening while the revered Charles Finney's white-floured head snowed gently on his honored collar.

Some students (ahem) succumbed at times to pride at the volume and depth of histories and poems and manifestos conquered in Mrs. Helms' class, but Peter's quiet, humble matching and outmatching of our efforts reminded us that it was a gift to sit at the feet of the ancients, and that we would all be held accountable for what we made of it.

We were blessed to be students of the Classics, and eventually we even admitted it. As Pastor Helms explained every year in his devotional accompaniment to the "Classics" lecture, we ought to study history because it is the record of the Creator's works. Those who are taught have a duty—to their peers, to their communities, to the next generation—to give what they have been given, to pass on beautiful works, world-shaping ideas, and most important, the Truth as echoed through eons-worth of classic works and ultimately in the one Book and its Mediator, the God-Man who laid down his life to rescue his people.

"What are you going to study in college, Heidi?"
"Classical studies, I think. Books and history—things like that."
"You like that kind of stuff?"
"I think it's beautiful."

Chapter Seven

The extreme greatness of Christianity lies in the fact that it does not seek a supernatural remedy for suffering, but a supernatural use for it.
—Simone Weil

One Saturday evening, about four weeks into Peter's hospital stay as I took my turn in his room, I had a surprise visit from the doctor who was head over the entire trauma unit. Around forty and just beginning to bald, he looked at me with professional concern when he tracked me down at the nurse's desk outside Peter's room. He said he'd heard we wanted to take Peter home. Was that true? I said it was and he looked downcast.

After a pause, he said quietly, "You do not know what this will be like. I don't want anyone to have sold you a bill of goods. Don't you know that you will end up tired and sick yourself and unable to care for Peter or for yourselves?"

Something in his tone made my head start to swim and feel very heavy. I sat down to keep from feeling faint. As he continued, I realized he was trying to prepare me for a worst-case kind of scenario, one in which Peter might stay like he was for years. He said again, "You don't know what this will be like."

At some point, his demeanor roused my pride. "Dr. Kadur," I said in a low voice, with all my might trying to cover the shakiness, "I am a full-time, stay-at-home mom. I have homeschooled my children since they were toddlers. My eldest son is now a doctoral student at Notre Dame University. My twenty-two-year-old son is an accountant and married. My daughter is a Texas All-State violinist, and Peter himself is a National Merit Finalist. He was on his way to a private university on academic scholarship this fall." I paused to help emphasize my final words. "I *know* what it is to invest in the lives of my children, and I am ready to invest in Peter now."

He looked at me. "Have you seen any response in him?" he asked softly. "We have seen some slight responsiveness," I answered.

With that, he entered Peter's room and approached his bedside. Leaning over, he spoke loudly, "Peter! Open your eyes!" Peter's eyes widened at once.

Then he looked at Peter's clenched hands and rigid arms, crossed over his chest. "Peter! Give me a thumbs up with your right hand!" Peter's left hand and thumb began to move.

"This thumb, Peter." I touched the right. His whole hand, along with his thumb, slowly lifted off his chest.

Dr. Kadur motioned me back into the hall. I asked him if he was more hopeful now. He nodded, a tentative look of relief on his face, and told me he wanted to meet with the whole family as soon as possible. I was to summon everyone I thought should be there.

Andrew, Caleb and Hope, and Beth were taking the Saturday afternoon off for a swim at Hope's parents' house. I called Doug and them and the grandparents and asked them to come to the hospital at once. The kids showed up in their swimsuits.

An hour later, Dr. Kadur met us in one of the hospital's family rooms, small and windowless with sofas and arm chairs. He brought a chaplain with him. He began with a summary of how far Peter had come in his recovery. The statistics were alarming: half of all brain-injured people die at the scene of the accident. Only 50 percent of those who make it to the hospital survive the first day. Of that diminishing number, half die during the first week. Of the fraction still alive after the first week, infections still claim many lives.

At the time, Peter was still receiving strong antibiotics. "So, you are saying we could still lose him to infection," Doug stated matter-of-factly.

"Yes," the doctor's solemn reply. We later found out that the overall survival rate for TBI (traumatic brain injury) as severe as Pete's was only about 10 percent.

He told us that the greatest thing we could give Peter right now was our love and support. He turned to Andrew and said, "The brain is like Darwin's black box. There's still so much we don't know about it. We know that people under age nineteen still have a lot of repair enzymes operating in their brains. So he has age on his side. Just go through his recovery with an attitude that no one knows what his recovery will be like, and don't get hung up on small details."

That night, I was still trembly at the fearful encounter. The likely long-term nature of Peter's injury and recovery began to dawn on me. And the question entered my mind, "Okay, Selah, if you had the choice of Peter dying and escaping the whole agonizing ordeal ahead with its ups, downs, and outrageous unknowns, or of Peter living, not knowing at all what it will look like or the toll it will take on your family, what would you choose?"

I considered only briefly. "You choose, Lord. I can't choose. You must be the One." And that was that.

I found out a few days later that Doug had experienced the exact same encounter with the Lord. He had answered the question just as I had.

On Facebook:

August 31, 2010
Saturday we had a consultation with the head doctor of the trauma unit. We learned that the small responses we have been seeing for at least the last week or so are signs that Peter has barely emerged from his coma. This is sobering, but the doctor told us that Peter has age on his side, and that in young people his age, the brain still has repair enzymes operating. He said the biggest thing is that Peter has a lot of family love and support in his favor. The doctor frankly admitted there was still much that is unknown about the brain and he can give us no certain prognosis. We voiced our confidence to him that Peter is in the hands of the Lord.

Now that Peter is emerging into consciousness, these are our prayer requests:

1. *That we would be able to mentally absorb a daunting volume of information on rehabilitation from traumatic brain injury.*
2. *That the Lord would cause each cell in Peter's brain to make new connections, spark new pathways, and regather old memories, and that Peter would have an abundance of those "repair enzymes" associated with his youth.*

For the family,
Hope

Chapter Seven

*August 29, 2010: A Great Cloud of Witnesses; A Message from Dad
Suffering is so alien to us. And we in the culture of the healthcare explosion and American prosperity end up so surprised when it visits us. We're kinda spoiled that way. I know I am. Some of my new heroes are those of you I have heard from who've borne heavy suffering so gracefully in the privacy of your own homes and lives.*

I have also drawn great comfort from older brothers and sisters who've gone before us, whose stories reveal that suffering makes itself familiar in lives where the Lord wants to reveal himself.

Let me introduce you to one of our older brothers, B.B. Warfield, a Christian from the nineteenth century. He described the tendency we Christians have to veer toward the one extreme or the other of either emphasizing a strong devotion to the Lord, but dismissing theology, or of holding to good teaching without a warm heart towards God. When we are tempted either to say, "Theology doesn't matter—I just love God," or to think that it's acceptable to have head knowledge and right thinking without warmhearted devotion, we are making a false dichotomy. Warfield described it as asking a soldier going into battle which leg he would like to take along. He must have both, without question.

These older saints tended to own a much more God-centered view of life than we do. Our religion has a lot of man-centeredness in it. These bygone saints knew that God is "the point," and not we ourselves. This enabled them to gracefully suffer many losses. Warfield himself married a beautiful young woman who was struck by lightning on their honeymoon. He cared for her as an invalid for almost forty years, cheerfully and quietly arranging his duties as a professor around her needs. They never had children.

Another older brother, Adoniram Judson, toiled away in Burma for years, losing to the strenuous living conditions some of his children, his first wife, his second wife, and his own good health. After years of labor, he had only won a scant handful of people to the Lord. Once, he got so discouraged that he meditated for days by an open grave. Yet he eventually returned to his work. The Lord used his efforts in the end to touch a whole tribe of thousands who had been waiting for the good news that they had been foretold would come. Today this group remains actively Christian in spite of severe persecution.

Our parents (or grandparents, for some of you) lived in the generation of Jim and Elisabeth Elliott. Jim and four other men went on mission to share Christ with a remote tribe along the Amazon. All five were killed before they had a chance to say one word about Christ. Jim's widow, Elisabeth, chose to live with the Auca Indians for a time to bring the gospel to the very people who had murdered her husband.

All of these were only able to endure the suffering that intruded into their lives when they held fast to the idea that God is in control and that God works for the good of his people through their suffering. They refused to look at second causes. They trusted that God moves all things forward for the purposes that he intends for our lives and for his kingdom on earth. He himself is the mover and shaker behind all events. Yet that thought caused no fear in their minds or mistrust of his goodness. Rather, this understanding freed them to love God because they were not focused on other people or Satan as causes. They looked to God alone.

And I do not have time to tell about Jonathan and Sarah Edwards, William Carey, Corrie ten Boom, Horatio Spafford, Joseph Scriven, Samuel Rutherford, and clouds of others, who by faith endured crippling losses under the hand of an Omnipotent God, and by love found firm stone pathways through waters of suffering. They created hymns from the depths; they left family legacies of unshakeable devotion; they won to Christ nations still zealous to this day. They beckon us to rediscover the solid footing as we cross those waters of suffering ourselves.

I'll conclude with a few words from Charles Spurgeon, who long battled health problems and depression, knowing that his beloved England was in the process of rejecting the gospel. Spurgeon left us much in the way of a strong theology and a warm heart toward God. Listen to what he says: "The God of Providence has limited the time, manner, intensity, repetition, and effects of all our sicknesses; each throb is decreed, each sleepless hour predestined, each relapse ordained, each depression of the spirit foreknown, and each sanctifying result eternally purposed. Nothing great or small escapes the ordaining hand of him who numbers the hairs of our head."

Doug

So Pete was going to walk a path through some deep waters of suffering. And we as his family would be walking along with him. The prognosis was frightening, and the temptation to despair overwhelming at times, but the Lord rescued me from such dark thoughts with assurances that he had given us much to make it easier. We began to see how we could minister to Peter, despite the extent of his future challenges. Throughout his seventeen years, the Lord had fashioned Peter into a determined young man, a quiet encourager. In exactly this way, we could now serve him. We would encourage the encourager; we would treat him as the man he'd become.

As physical therapists and nurses came and went from Peter's room, giving us crash courses on various aspects of home health care, I reflected on Peter's childhood. Andrew and I found ourselves discussing what a blessing Peter had been to our family over the years. He was a steady and consistent encourager to each one of us. I guess it somewhat inadvertently began way back when Pete was a toddler and a frequent tag-along to his older siblings. He'd smile, wave, and cheer them on at soccer games, violin lessons, and recitals.

As he got older, Peter explored his own activities: Scouts, basketball, piano, speech and debate. He had his own life, was secure in himself. But he never outgrew the role of family encourager.

So when Andrew moved up to Indiana to attend Notre Dame, Peter drove up with him to move all his stuff. He was out front as the family member keeping in closest touch with his brother, making sure Andrew didn't forget what an important part of the family he was even though far away. When Caleb was making plans for marriage, Peter helped him prepare his new home for his bride. And when Beth went "off" to college, but kept living at home, Peter pitched in to do her chores along with his own at those frequent times when she felt weighted down with homework.

It was the same way with his parents and his church family. After his accident, all sorts of jobs had to be filled by others — things many of us weren't even aware that Peter had been quietly taking care of: printing and folding bulletins early Sunday mornings, helping clean the church building, frying up Saturday breakfast with Doug for the men's book studies (he never complained about not getting to sleep in on these Saturdays). His service reached many others in our church family; his broad shoulders had helped move a number of households.

Chapter Seven

I remember thinking that Peter was like a classically educated Samwise Gamgee (from *The Lord of the Rings*). He was always quietly helping someone else succeed. He was brave when we were weak. He was loyal when we were discouraged. And when we were fatigued, he helped shoulder our burden. He also happened to be a National Merit Finalist—a really smart kid. Confirming our own experiences, reports of Pete's servant heart trickled in from others as well:

Dear Helms family,
Peter made a strong impression on us during the speech tournaments. My son, Jonathan, debated him several times. Peter has such a kind and loving way, and radiates the love of the Lord! We have been praying for you all and will continue. The Lord Jesus is sufficient to bring you through this!

With love and concern,
The Paul Drumwright family

Just today, our daughters Maggie and Janna recalled the kindness Peter (a senior at the time, and the girls, freshmen) demonstrated during what was a very challenging academic course for them: "We always made sure to be in Peter's discussion group. He always took the time to listen to our opinions and made us feel like we were significant and that our thoughts were valid." This gift of encouragement is, among so many other traits Peter displays, such a rare and precious gift. This is the person for whom we pray, and whom the Lord so loves. He continues to give to us, even in his present weakness.
Martha Elisabeth Walker

This was one of the graces God gave our family: it was not at all hard to think of serving Peter in his present weakness. It's always a blessing to get to serve one who has offered himself in service to the Lord and to others. Over the years and with a sense of awe and privilege, our family had gladly hosted missionaries, preachers, and humble servants of the Lord. Paul himself reminded the Philippians of the honor of serving men like Epaphroditus. Just as Peter had served the Lord by modeling as much Christian service as a young man of seventeen could show, it was easy for us to serve the Lord by serving Peter. Overwhelming thoughts often crowded in regarding what this injury might mean for Peter and for us. My worry over how difficult it could prove to be rose to intense levels at times. But, as a family, we decided that when the Lord opened the door for us to care for Peter at home, we must view it as an unspeakable privilege. Jesus told us plainly, "But not so with you. Rather, let the greatest among you become as the youngest, and the leader as one who serves.... I am among you as one who serves." This understanding of Peter as an imperfect but stalwart young man of Christ helped to keep us faithful, as my post below described.

On Facebook:

September 1, 2010: Pete's a Man; A Message from Mom
There are other aspects to Peter than his literary, artistic side. He completed his Eagle Scout project the day before his car accident. He had overseen the construction of a chain-link fence, along with a timber and mulch perimeter, around our church's new playground.

Chapter Seven

He has strong opinions regarding politics. Several weeks ago, he had an intense discussion with his dad that went something like this: "Dad, I don't get it. All of these conservative Tea Party people are talking about the possibility of revolution because of the financial situation of the country. I know that high taxes are immoral and worth a strong backlash. But I don't get why we conservatives are so outraged about taxes when we haven't revolted because of abortion. Abortion is a much greater evil than high taxes. I feel like we are being hypocrites. If we would really revolt about taxes, we should've put up a fight years ago over abortion." He was pretty much ready to take up arms.

His more level-headed dad reviewed our family discussions about which wars throughout history were "just" wars, and how that must be determined. Were all other lesser means exhausted? Is it a last resort? Can it be declared by a proper authority who would have a just cause? Would it put innocent lives in danger? Would the end be proportionate to the means used? And so on. I'm not sure he changed Pete's mind on it.

When Peter has faced challenges with school and friends during his high school years, he has assumed an attitude of "What does the Lord want to teach me through this?" and "How should I grow through this?" On his own initiative, he has registered for several biblical counseling seminars—just to encourage his own spiritual walk and to inform himself for ministry. He is a biblically directed guy.

He once referred to himself to Doug and me as our "jock son," (much to Caleb's objection). He enjoys a sweaty game of pickup basketball with his friends or a round of soccer with the Rock Creek "kids" (ages five to seventy-three) after our Wednesday fellowship meal and prayer.

So, as were preparing to bring Peter home from the hospital, Doug came to us as a family one day. He told us that, though our hearts were breaking, we should resist the temptation to feel sorry for Pete. He told us, "Remember, Pete is a man. We need to think of him as one." He wrote that day: "I have less temptation to feel sorry for my son, because I have seldom seen him mired in self-pity. He has always been a trooper through tough times, and that makes it easier to see his suffering as a divine calling rather than a horrible tragedy. We are not victims, we are victors in Christ!"

I confess that when I had been visiting Pete's bedside, I had been calling him "Sweetie," and other such Mom-like terms. But Andrew took the cue from his dad. "You're a good soldier, Pete. Be brave. We are plugging for you."

Once, a woman from our church had Peter and some others help her son with a project. She observed Peter's spirit in the face of slow, not very fruitful labor. "Peter's so much like his father," she said, ". . . quiet, steadfast, tenacious." May the Lord give him the tenacity of young manliness now.

"Have I not commanded you? Be strong and courageous. Do not be frightened, and do not be dismayed, for the Lord your God is with you wherever you go." Joshua 1:9

Selah

September 7, 2010: Update
The doctors have been in the process of weaning Peter off his trach. They put in a new trach over the weekend and there have been a lot of secretions

from Pete's lungs. He has not been very responsive since they made this change. It has been pretty difficult on his body. The doctors recommended he stay in the hospital until he can go home trach-free, and we are comfortable with that.

Thank you.

For the family,
Hope

Chapter 8

The great thing, if one can, is to stop regarding all the unpleasant things as interruptions of one's "own," or "real" life. The truth is of course that what one calls the interruptions are precisely one's real life – the life God is sending one day by day: what one calls one's "real life" is a phantom of one's own imagination. —C.S. Lewis

Our goal by this time was to bring Peter home and care for him there until he woke up enough to enter a formal rehab program. No one could tell us how long that would take. We were learning enough in the hospital to recognize when someone wasn't getting some aspect of his nursing care right. Surely we now knew enough to do this at home. Some doctors were skeptical of our ability to do this; others were sure we could, given the support Peter had. One thing we knew for sure—Doug and I had grown very weary of passing each other in the parking lot on our way in and out of the hospital; we hoped to get some of our life back now that it was several weeks post-accident.

Chapter 8

On Facebook:

September 9, 2010: A New World; A Message from Mom
Until a few weeks ago, we used to have church visitors over for lunch on Sundays. I greatly enjoyed discipling the younger women at our church. And I was busy collecting boxes to pack up Peter's dishes and such before he headed off to college. On the verge of an "empty nest," I was also looking towards finishing up my certification for a biblical counseling training course.

Life today is very different, as you might imagine.

I was trying to explain to a good friend the other day what hospital life is like after so long. I'll tell you as well: it's like going to a new world every day. I mean, like through a wardrobe door. And, Narnia-style, every day in a hospital is like a thousand years. There is so much that happens. It's strenuous. People fight for their lives. You see sights and hear sounds that you never knew in the old world. There are desperate battles going on for your soul. You meet strangers who become friends and who will fight for you. You watch your loved one struggle to overcome his archenemy, and you hope to hold a healing flask of oil to bring him back to you when he falls. There are mazes of paperwork to add to the obstacles in your path. And they keep it frigid in there—it's always winter.

And then, finally, whenever you exit the hospital doors (back through the wardrobe) and drive away, you find that only five minutes have passed in the old world of home. There are still dishes that need to be washed, laundry that needs to be folded, and bills that need to be paid, just as when you left home that morning, a thousand years ago.

When you are in the old world, you find that no one really can understand what has happened to you and how it has changed you, unless you can find someone who has also been transported into that same world via the wardrobe door and has fought the same battles. It can be quite unsettling.

And really, as a pastor's wife and homeschooling mom, I am accustomed to have unexpected new assignments that were not necessarily of my own planning or inclination. The hardest part about this newest task is missing Peter's voice and fellowship. And the unknown.

There is really only one remedy for this difficulty. And that is the work of the Lion of the tribe of Judah. He's not safe at all. But he's good. And he will make us serviceable to him, which is really what he has intended all along. He never meant for us to be addicted to our own personal peace and prosperity. He has stuff for us to do.

> "Wrong will be right, when Aslan comes in sight,
> At the sound of his roar, sorrows will be no more,
> When he bares his teeth, winter meets its death,
> And when he shakes his mane, we shall have spring again."
> – C.S. Lewis in The Lion, the Witch, and the Wardrobe.

"It will be said on that day, 'Behold, this is our God; we have waited for him, that he might save us. This is the Lord; we have waited for him; let us be glad and rejoice in his salvation.'" Isaiah 25:9

Selah

Chapter 8

Over a year later, we received a response to this post from another mother who had experienced much the same struggle:

Your son is dear to our hearts! We have been in prayer for Peter since last year when a friend shared your post comparing the daily hospital visits with entering Narnia. How profound that post was, as our son was ill and required daily visits for nearly three months and other doctor visits over the past year. Life is very fragile and how God uses all of it for his glory is so humbling.

I am thankful that you penned those words as I could not adequately communicate to others exactly how our world had been changed, even though the other world carried on. Who we met, what we saw, conversations we had, with both fellow Christians and nonbelievers, so many in the fight for their lives, will be forever etched in our minds. A richness, a depth to our son and all of our family came about through tremendous heartache. How can that be? I know it doesn't make sense. But we have been to Narnia and are changed because of it. And I know that our Father in heaven will use all of it, all of what Peter and your family is going through, all of what our son and our family is going through for His good.

Tender blessings,
The Blacks

Every day, the respiratory therapist gave Peter a challenge in which they capped off the airway to his trach, forcing him to breathe through his nose. He had difficulty doing this at first, but began to make progress. We hoped Pete would continue to make steps forward in this area so we could bring him home, but we didn't know for sure why he was having such difficulty breathing without the trach. Perhaps Peter's neck muscles were so weak that he couldn't keep his airway open in order to breathe through his throat. Or maybe he just wasn't conscious enough to hold his head straight.

Because of this slow trach-weaning process, we didn't know exactly when we would be bringing Peter home. Hospital schedules often change and we were learning to be flexible.

On Facebook:

September 18, 2010
Last week the doctors did a CT scan to see why Peter had been set back so much after the second trach was put in. We found out that the trach was actually too big and was pressing on a major artery. They changed it immediately and Pete is now back on track towards coming home! He continues to be given breathing challenges where they cap the trach and allow him to breathe through his airway for as long as he can.

On Tuesday, Dad and Mom are planning to meet with doctors from another hospital to discuss some possibilities for the next stage of Peter's care. We hope that we will be able to get the family trained and better prepared to bring him home.

Thank you!
Hope

Chapter 8

While we spent our days at the hospital learning how to care for Peter, hoping to get him home, Dr. Kadur quietly advocated for us behind the scenes. Slowly it became apparent that getting Peter off the trach quickly was an overly ambitious goal. So Dr. Kadur stepped in, knowing how staggering it would be for us to shoulder nursing care, plus trach care, plus TBI therapy, all at home. Word trickled down to us through the nurses that Dr. Kadur was negotiating with Baylor Institute of Rehabilitation to admit us for an intensive two-week training. Though the trauma hospital had taught us a lot about caring for an invalid, the Baylor program would fine-tune our understanding of therapy for someone with brain injury and give us a greater comfort level for doing optimum home care. Things began to happen quickly.

On Facebook:

September 25, 2010
Here are the things that you can pray for:

1. *That the family will be rested, available, healthy, and attentive, so that we can absorb a mountain of information and training.*
2. *That the doctor will be able to quickly intuit Peter's condition and will have wisdom on the best course to pursue for him. (We've understood that every individual has a unique path to recovery and that no "cookie cutter" mold works for all patients.)*
3. *That Peter will progress in becoming more conscious as a result of the rehab center's cutting edge methodologies. So far, his responses include finding us or an object with his eyes, and*

gripping our hands strongly. He appears to be working on other responses as well.

4. *That the Lord would continue to refire neurons and connections in Peter's brain and that much healing could take place in a short stretch of time. We've heard of instances where, with the right stimulation, parts of an injured brain can suddenly "kick in" and resume function quickly.*
5. *Continue to pray that Peter will be medically stable and soon be trach-free. His trach challenges are continuing to progress slowly.*

Over the next couple weeks, updates might be even sparser as our family undergoes the training at Baylor. However, we will do our best to keep you updated with Peter's condition and our prayer concerns as we journey ahead.

Thank you all for your support and prayers.

For the family,
Hope

So Dr. Kadur eventually arranged it so that we would take Peter to Baylor so that his family could receive this invaluable two-week training in caring for him at home until he was ready for strenuous inpatient rehab. Dr. Kadur had paved our way by telling Baylor all about Peter and our commitment to him. We would learn from Margaret Carrington, one of the best rehab doctors in the country. "The brain responds to stimulation," we'd been hearing since Pete's accident. So we were ready to absorb

Chapter 8

all manner of information about how we could help jumpstart his brain's ability to knit its neuro-fibers back together. So Doug and I, Caleb and Hope, Andrew, Beth, and Gramma Helms moved into a small apartment in North Dallas for the two weeks that we would be there. The whole family would be in on all the learning.

We checked in the following Monday to begin our round-the-clock training. Dr. Carrington spent more time poring over Peter on his first afternoon at Baylor than all the doctors combined throughout the eight weeks Peter had been at the trauma hospital. Focused, thorough, deliberate, she talked to Peter and tried to get him to make eye contact with her and to give her a thumbs up. Straightaway, she gave him a new trach, and he immediately began to breathe more comfortably.

"I'm hopeful," she told us that day. "A young man with that much brain could afford to lose some and still have some left over."

She continued to check in on him every morning, sometimes very early, attentive to his every move, studying, noting. One morning she told Doug, "You know, I really think he's going to pull out of this."

She related the story of a young motorcycle racer. One day while racing his motorcycle at one hundred miles per hour, he had run into a brick wall. All he could do for a year was move his eyes and look around. Today, she said, he was talking, texting, just newly walking, and he had a Facebook account up and going.

"I see more in Peter already than that young man had for a long time." That assurance alone was worth our trip there. Then she looked at me meaningfully. "And I have learned that, with people of faith, whatever happens will be good."

The first Sunday morning of Peter's stay, I saw Dr. Carrington working at the front desk, and I stopped to chat. She mentioned

Peter's National Merit standing and the fact that he was homeschooled. She expressed admiration. I told her that Doug and I had never set out to make "intellectuals" of our children. Rather, we had taught them that God made the world and that God made them—both for his own glory. And God is at work in his world. This understanding gave them a love for life and learning. Peter's intellect was only a by-product. I told her that though we were proud of Peter's achievements, mainly we just missed *him* because he is such an important part of our family and so dear to us. She smiled.

Over the next few days, things began to happen. Medical staff filed into Peter's room continually, having heard about us. They asked Andrew if he was the one from Notre Dame. They told us that Dr. Carrington was trying to get Botox injections for Peter's jaws and arms to help them relax from the muscle contractions characteristic to TBI patients. They told us that when Dr. Carrington goes after something, she usually gets it.

One morning, she entered Pete's room and told us she'd been thinking about our stories of Peter all weekend and couldn't get him off her mind. She asked if the hospital administrator had come to Peter's room. She had told him, "You need to go down and meet that family. It will restore your faith in humankind and in the ability of parents to raise good kids in this world."

She asked more questions about homeschooling. "Did you and your husband teach them all they know?" No, the Lord provided them opportunities to sit under many people with varying expertise. And sometimes we just knew what the goal was and learned along with them.

The following Friday, four doctors appeared in Peter's room—Margaret Carrington's recruits. She hoped they would bless Peter

Chapter 8

with procedures and injections that would alleviate all manner of brain injury side effects. They all greeted us warmly. After the procedures were completed, Dr. Carrington and her assistant followed up with us in Peter's room. She told me that these doctors had rendered their services free of charge and apologized that hospital protocol required her to send us a bill for her own.

"Oh, but you have given so much already," I said. As a thank you, I gave her a color copy of one of Peter's pencil sketches from the *Star-Telegram* stock show art contest, along with an envelope full of posts from the PRAY FOR PETER HELMS Facebook group. She thanked me and hugged me warmly. She said she was decorating her Oklahoma retirement home with a western theme, and that Pete's print would enjoy a prominent place there.

I asked her and her assistant if they would like to see Peter performing in his most recent piano recital (Grampa had posted a recording of it online). They said they would. As Grampa's title appeared, "Peter Helms plays Rachmaninoff," Dr. Carrington drew close to the screen. "Oh, I love Rachmaninoff!" Then the credits showed the piece, "Prelude in C# minor." And she exclaimed, "That's my favorite piece of music in all the world. My father was a classical pianist, and he played that piece."

She turned to her assistant. "Do you know how hard that piece is? Is he playing it from memory?" She questioned back at me. I nodded.

As he appeared on the screen, I said, "That's our son, Peter."

"How long ago was this?" the assistant inquired.

"It was in May, just four months ago," I replied. Her eyes filled with tears.

I didn't see Dr. Carrington again till Monday morning. She was coming out of the café area, and I followed her onto the elevator.

I greeted her, and she asked how Peter's phenol injections had affected his ankles and feet. We chatted briefly, and she said, "You know I really liked reading those writings and getting to know Peter better. I really liked the one where you told how he helps fry up breakfast for your men's meetings at church."

"Yes, nothing big or amazing, just small and quiet acts of service. That's Peter." I said.

"I want you to know," she continued, "that I, like you, consider it a privilege to serve Peter." Then she reiterated her admiration for our family.

"Well, no strength in us accomplishes anything," I said. "We get our strength from the Lord, and he is our life."

She thanked me again for the posts and the drawing, and I said that I hoped they would make us friends. As we walked into Peter's room, she repeated to Doug, who had been waiting there, the privilege it had been for her to serve Peter. She called him her best patient ever. Doug gave her a hug. Then I hugged her, and she kissed me on the cheek.

Early in our stay, she had told me that if she'd had children of her own, she would definitely choose to homeschool them now that she knew more about it. The day we'd arrived, she told us that she received every patient into her facility as they were and tried to bring them to the next level of their potential. How like mothering was this! It struck me how this sixty-ish woman, a respected professional in her field, had channeled all the nurturing instincts of her feminine nature into the lives of her TBI patients. Baylor is one of the top twenty rehabilitation programs in the country, and we received a lot of great training from the specialists there. As head of the program, Dr. Carrington was truly a gift from God.

Chapter 8

Her great skill and knowledge combined with a great amount of compassion and personal devotion to each of her patients.

While Peter was at Baylor, he was given various neurostimulants to help him progress toward fully waking up. His ability to track movement with his eyes improved substantially, but we still waited eagerly for the rest of his body to follow commands. When Pete could consistently follow commands and track with his eyes, he would be ready for rehab.

On Facebook:

October 4, 2010: Update
Right now Peter is still unready for rehab, so we will be working with him at home on the things the specialists have been teaching us. We have received great training from the occupational therapists, physical therapists, speech therapists, and a neuropsychologist. We hope to bring Peter home in a week or so when we are done with our training.

Right now Pete has some responsiveness and we are hopeful that it will increase as the weeks and months pass, but his responsiveness is still pretty minimal and there is no way of knowing if he's being intentional until he can communicate with us. Right now we are working with him on basic responses, such as trying to get him to swallow so he can manage his secretions and doing anything we can that might stimulate his body to remember the things he used to do.

It was easy to be impatient for Pete to "wake up" completely. But we learned that consciousness is a lot more complicated than we first thought. It is not always a matter of being either awake or in a coma. When explaining Peter's situation, it's easier to think of consciousness as a scale with the left of the scale being total unresponsiveness, and the other end normal function. Peter was diagnosed as "minimally conscious." He was not vegetative and could respond to some commands occasionally. Using a Rancho Scale of 0 (comatose) to 8 (fully conscious, normal responses), Baylor diagnosed Peter at a Level 3.

After two weeks, Peter arrived home to a nervous but grateful family. His care would be managed by Doug, Gramma, Andrew, Beth, and me. Now we would continue the program begun at Baylor and the therapy they creatively designed to bring Peter's life back to him and to us. God's people were there to help; on the day he returned, six loving people worked full time to get Peter's home-care off the ground.

The doctors were all very hopeful that being at home could give him further comfort and the stimulation that he required to become more conscious. He needed to smell Dad's eggs and bacon frying in the mornings and to hear the clink of Scout's dog tag on her collar. He needed to see familiar faces around the dining table where he'd eaten all his life, Doug coming in the front door in the evenings, Beth and me washing dishes or getting supper in the oven. And as we watched over him, he seemed really relaxed and comfortable in the intimate surroundings.

On Facebook:

October 6, 2010: Members of One Another

Chapter 8

I love the Lord's people. Peter's injury has truly shaken our world and has been draining and grueling, but we've found immense comfort in the family of the Lord. Let me share with you just a tiny handful of the blessings we've received.

One godly gentleman showed up at the hospital a little more than a week ago, having just arrived from Virginia. (We are in Texas.) He and his wife talked with Doug and me in the hospital waiting room for a bit, then he asked to go back and pray for Peter in his room. After he'd knelt and asked the Lord to heal our son, he stood and said to Peter, "Peter, we traveled all this way so that I could come in here and pray with you."

Believers we have never met have written us the most beautiful cards and notes describing their urgent and frequent prayers for our son. They saturate their cards with Scripture and hymns that breathe life to our souls.

One man posted on the group wall: "Peter and family, you now have some really fine people in Mexico City who are praying for you – young Mexican nationals who are dedicated, serving Christians. I pray that some day soon you will all get to visit together because I know you will love each other! May God grant it."

One young woman told us that she was pretty sure almost the whole state of Arizona was praying for Peter. Another woman I hadn't seen in forty years (I had known her in my childhood) traveled to the hospital from out of town to reassure us of her prayers for Peter. I've had Christian moms from several states tell me that their three-year-olds remind them throughout the day to pray for Peter.

Doug cashed a check at a local bank last week. A man came out and introduced himself as the president of the bank and asked, "Are you Pastor Helms?" Doug said he was, and the man told him that everyone at that bank was praying for Peter. Of many instances I could mention, these are only a sampling.

The really deep chord that sounds in all this is an amazing harmony among God's people because his Spirit indwells us. We love each other and pray for each other because of that Spirit we all share. We see his life in each other, and it makes us happy and attached to one another. It strikes me forcefully that it is the Lord who lays individual, hurting believers on our hearts for prayer. And if the Lord has laid Peter on the hearts of all of you, it is to reveal that he loves Peter and is working for his good. It comforts me tremendously to know that he is urging you precious believers to pray for our son. What a great revelation of his love for Peter!

But Peter's situation isn't unique in all this. These are only noteworthy instances of what happens any time we sense that another believer has walked into the room, bringing with him a grace and a oneness that allows us to recognize the Spirit of Christ. We feel a kinship with him (just like you feel with Peter), and we want to respond to him and pray for his needs. (Perhaps it's a bit like what the two disciples felt on the road to Emmaus when their hearts leapt within them, even though they thought they were speaking to an ordinary man.) It's the Spirit of the Lord recognizing and loving the Spirit of the Lord. How the Lord is glorified when we love each other; there is a unity of communion within his own character and presence.

It's a great comfort to walk through life with the Lord's people . . . who become his vessels to spill onto each other his own Spirit.

Chapter 8

"May the God of endurance and encouragement grant you to live in such harmony with one another, in accord with Christ Jesus, that together you may with one voice glorify the God and Father of our Lord Jesus Christ."
Romans 15:5,6

Selah

Chapter 9

And as I read, an incredible thought prickled the back of my neck. Was it possible that this — all of this that seemed so wasteful and so needless — this war, Scheveningen prison, this very cell — none of it was unforeseen or accidental? Could it be part of the pattern first revealed in the Gospels? Hadn't Jesus... been defeated as utterly and unarguably as our little group and our small plans had been? But...if the Gospels were truly the pattern of God's activity, then defeat was only the beginning. I would look around the bare little cell and wonder what conceivable victory could come from a place like this.
— Corrie ten Boom

The night before Peter's transfer to Baylor, we received a phone call from Doug's sister, Anita. A young man in their church, Daniel Heinrich, had been struck and killed by a drunk driver while on his way to witness in downtown Fort Worth. Anita had just received a phone call from Daniel's mom at the scene of the accident.

But Daniel and Peter were only the first two.

Later that same month, a young man from a neighboring community sustained a brain aneurysm as he and his younger brother

Chapter 9

drove down a local freeway. His brain incident caused a car wreck that gave him a double brain injury—first from the aneurysm, and then from the trauma. He also came from a Christian family. I heard about it from a nurse with the home healthcare group that had come to help with Peter. We knew people from the church that he and his family attended. We followed his story on the Caringbridge site as he spent about seventy days in a coma very similar to Peter's. He also contracted an infection. The infection eventually claimed his life.

Another young man from a Bible church in Fort Worth also died in a car accident.

So tightly knit is our Christian community in Fort Worth that most of us either knew these young men personally or knew someone who knew them. Then, in the midst of this upsetting local news, our daughter-in-law, Hope, showed up at our home one day with the news that friends of her family from Arkansas had just lost their two teenaged boys on a single day in a freak car accident.

We began to feel like a communal Rachel weeping for her children who were no more. What was happening to the next generation of young men—young men equipped and willing to be leaders for our future? No words satisfy.

We didn't have the answer. Yet, in our grief, we reached out to each other. Daniel's mother and sister came to my home to help me organize our medical supplies for Peter. Doug attended a gathering at a mutual friend's house and ended up in a conversation with Daniel's father. They bolstered each other's faith, drawing on the theology that would sustain them through this puzzling time.

One bereaved mom came to my home to do laundry, freeing me up to concentrate more on Peter's needs. Those first few weeks,

I couldn't clasp her closely enough as I listened to her relate her recent immersion in the fiery school of suffering.

"Selah," she told me, "I had been reading your posts on Peter's Facebook page all along, but I never knew they were preparing me for my own loss. I know what you mean when you say God's people have helped you face Peter's struggle. I feel I would be in an insane asylum without the support of God's people."

After my long weeks engaged in the struggle for Peter's life, her assessment applied equally to me.

"Our pastor told me, 'go ahead and cry. Just don't hole up,'" she said. "'In your sorrow, move out to invest in other people. Cry, and then go out and serve,' was the advice he gave," she said. "I am trying to do that."

And her sister Selah was a grateful beneficiary of that valiant spirit.

On Facebook:

October 23, 2010: A Message from Mom
"Why would the Lord allow a godly young man to be 'knocked out of commission' when there are already so few of them?" An honest question, asked by a young father who came to visit Peter in the hospital during the early weeks of his coma.

I'm sure many in Fort Worth were asking that very question three weeks ago when another seventeen-year-old young man, Daniel Heinrich, was struck and killed by a drunk driver while on his way to share the Gospel in downtown Fort Worth. This was a great blow to our sister churches in Fort Worth: two godly young men, Daniel and Peter, felled as they

Chapter 9

traveled toward ministry. Though Daniel and Peter did not know each other personally, they had many mutual friends among our community of believers—teenagers who marveled and grieved at the two events, so close together.

I can't say that I know all the reasons the Lord would allow these two accidents to happen, both so near in vicinity and timing and circumstances to the other. But I call to mind a story that gives me great hope. In Through Gates of Splendor, *Elisabeth Elliot tells of the martyrdom of five godly young men on the same day, her husband Jim Elliott and four other missionaries who were speared to death along the banks of the Curaray River, deep in the heart of the Amazon jungle. What a loss to the kingdom! Had they been protected from harm, one wonders, what amount of good might they have done for the cause of missions, the kingdom of God, and for their own children and grandchildren?*

But events of the past fifty years may help us not to second guess the Lord on such matters. Ask almost any retired missionary if he or anyone on his field of service landed there because of the influence of these five men. In the aftermath of Elliot's martyrdom, thousands of young people, now elderly, were inspired to join him and his friends in the cause of Christ. Even in the present generation, no small number serve Christ on the mission field in part due to the sacrifice made by Elliot and his friends. Heaven only will reveal the fruit that multiplied throughout history from their deaths.

For the godly man, neither his life, nor his life circumstances are ever "wasted." Not for Peter, and certainly not for Daniel. May the young people who have known these two be inspired to life-long service by their examples!

Further, think of the comfort to us parents, knowing that these two young men belong so surely to Christ. They have undoubtedly lived more abundantly in the seventeen or eighteen years they've been given than many do in seventy years and more. Life must be lived well every moment we are given, because no one knows how long he or she will have. How could this be shown any more clearly than through these circumstances?

Finally, as my dear husband reminds me, no matter how long we have to go without Peter's smile and fellowship, no matter how long life's sufferings last, if we stay the course and trust and obey in the old-fashioned way, Heaven will open to us as an eternal, beautiful day. On that day, our suffering will only seem to have lasted five minutes.

"Truly, truly, I say to you, unless a grain of wheat falls into the earth and dies, it remains alone; but if it dies, it bears much fruit." John 12:24

Selah

October 25, 2010: Update
It has been nice to have Peter home with us. We have put Peter's hospital bed in the living room so that he can be a part of our family activities and hear familiar sounds that might stimulate brain activity. Just this past week we celebrated Caleb's birthday, and we will be celebrating two more birthdays this week there in the living room with Peter.

Since being home, Pete has been able to follow objects with his eyes more (although not consistently), and has been doing better with his oral secretions by swallowing more. We try to utilize the things we learned at Baylor by doing things with Pete that will stimulate his brain. When we do actions with him that simulate what used to be familiar body movements, it is supposed to help his brain make new connections and, in time, send those signals on its own.

Please continue to pray for healing in Peter's brain, that he would be able to come to the next level of consciousness where he is able to respond consistently to simple commands, and that Pete will soon be trach-free. It would be a great blessing and so much more comfortable for Pete!

For the family,
Hope

We received messages from hundreds of people during these weeks offering support and hints that God was busy ripening much fruit on the vine of tragedy. Here are a few:

I've been checking this site almost daily. . . . It must be only by God's grace that both of you (and your families) are enduring the daily ordeals that you are facing. I think of Paul saying, "We are afflicted in every way, but not crushed; perplexed, but not despairing . . . ." God is obviously calling you to a higher level of faith than you ever had before—and certainly by a way you would never have chosen. But that's how heroes are made. And you have become that to me. So has Peter. Both of you have given him a strong spiritual foundation to get him through such a time as this. Somewhere inside that injured body and patient spirit, I know God is pouring his grace and whispering his love to him, every day, every moment.

Mark Mosher

We lifted Peter up before the LORD last night at Garner Baptist Church, and we will continue to do so. God is working in a lot of people's lives through this. May he be glorified and your precious family comforted and strengthened as only he can do.
Jill Cross

Peter, from Baghdad, Iraq, I'm still praying for your recovery. You will know one day soon that people have been praying for you from all corners of this world for a long time and are not giving up. God has his own timeline and purpose, and we don't or can't understand it oftentimes until way after the fact, maybe not even in this short life on earth. I've met you before and know that you are extremely bright and one of the few godly men in this corrupt, broken, and sick world. God must surely have a reason for this situation as he is in total control. I do believe that. May God heal you soon, according to his plan.
Ted Salazar

Selah, thank you for another powerful message of the faithfulness of God. Your and Doug's lives are such an example of the beauty of a Christ-likeness that is forged on the anvil of the Refiner's fire. You and your family have helped me in my walk with the Lord. Mary Jeanne and I are continually praying . . .
Charlie Hopkins

Oh my goodness . . . I joined this group soon after it was made, as a lot of my friends know Peter. I just now made the connection that Pastor Doug and the rest of the family used to visit my grandma, Ruby Cooper, who lived next door to me. She used to go to your church until she could no longer get out of the house. I don't know if you remember this, but when you visited, my parents, Joshua, Daniel, and I would go next door

Chapter 9

and we'd always fellowship and pray together. Brother Doug also did my grandma's funeral. Your family has always been such a blessing to mine. I just want you to know that my whole family has been praying for you all during this time. Thank you for everything, and God bless.

Betsy Cooper

We have loved the video clips of Peter playing piano, as well as the photo of his artwork. Thank you for sharing those! We continue to pray for his total healing and for your strength and stamina. So glad to hear he is home! I just visited my parents' church in St. Louis, and Peter was being prayed for there—has been on their prayer list for these many weeks. Many people asked about him and were so happy to hear he is now at home. They will continue to lift him (and your whole family) up to the Lord!

Sandra Ellman

Praise the LORD. God hears our prayer, knows the needs, and one day, God will open that door Peter is sitting behind to heal the brain cells and out will come Peter, the young man so many people have come to know and love without laying an eye on Peter. This is a witness to all who have heard about Peter and this family. . . .

Carrie Davis

Chapter 10

My dear brother, let God make of you what he will, he will end all with consolation, and shall make glory out of your sufferings; and would ye wish better work? —Samuel Rutherford

We threw our hearts into caring for Peter at home that month. It was good that he could be in a place so comfortable for him. We dragged the family's small black lab up into his lap, where she licked his face in welcome. She'd been a strong presence in Pete's childhood. We read books to him dating back to his early school years—from Paul Revere to the Pevensie kids. We played his favorite Hans Zimmer movie soundtracks and ran his fingers over his basketball.

Although Peter made some small improvements, he didn't show as much responsiveness as we had hoped. There were days he seemed much more alert watching us and "closer to the surface," but then he would drift away again—back "under" for a few days. A homeschool friend of mine, also a nurse, described it this way: sometimes he would seem as if he were in deep water, twenty feet below the surface and far away from us; other times he would be very near, as if he were just about to break the surface and come up out of the water. It reminded us that his healing was still more in the acute recovery stage, as we were told when we left Baylor.

After a month at home, another call from Baylor brought a change of plans. Baylor informed us that Peter had been approved for ankle surgery and a thirty-day stay in its rehab program. It's common for TBI patients to experience muscle contractures that cause their appendages to lock in one position, usually turned in or down. Pete's ankles had likewise contracted even though we were giving him daily physical therapy. We were grateful he would get this surgery so that one day, Lord willing, he would be able to walk again. We were told the surgery would be pretty simple, as it would involve clipping the Achilles tendon. Peter was moved to Baylor that afternoon. Hope posted a prayer update.

On Facebook:

November 10, 2010
Here are the things you can pray for:

1. *That the Lord would bring Peter to the point of consistent command following before our discharge date of December 10, because then he could just stay there and continue formal rehabilitation.*
2. *That the Lord would continue to heal his brain. The doctor did a new CT scan last week, and said that though his brain looks better, there are still bleeding and swelling issues.*
3. *That the family would have strength and trust in the Lord. This is a long, slow, roller coaster ride, and we sometimes can't help but battle weariness on every level. Pray that we could get some*

rest while Peter is in the hospital and we are not the ones doing all of his care.
4. That the Lord would give the therapists and doctors wisdom and good intuition about the best course for Peter. Practicing medicine for brain trauma is much more an art than a science, and there are a lot of variables that go into deciding treatment for each individual. Sometimes it is just a matter of trying out different medications and therapies to see what works for a particular patient. It would be neat if the Lord would show them the best thing for Peter on first trial.

For the family,
Hope

Everyone at Baylor exclaimed over how good Peter looked and how much more alert he appeared since his discharge in October.

Pete's tracking was stronger and more consistent. He could endure longer therapy sessions, and he seemed to be responding more to simple commands: opening his mouth, swallowing (at times), and giving thumbs up. He still did not respond to commands often enough to be called "consistent," but one of the doctors told us that his bad days during this stay at Baylor were better than his good days during the last. In fact, Peter's ratings on the neuropsychologist's scale of assessment in October had been consistently in "near coma" range. When we returned in November, he scored in the "no coma" range a few times. So the overall trajectory indicated continued improvement, for which we were grateful.

The occupational therapists bounced Pete around in a sitting position on therapy balls. This helped stimulate his body's internal

Chapter 10

systems and strengthen his core muscles. They propped him up on his elbows, explaining to us that stress on major joints triggers deep muscle memories. One day while they were working with him, we actually heard his voice for the first time since his accident. These spontaneous sounds did not take the form of actual words, but thrilled us nonetheless. Pete also made attempts to hold up his head, though he tired very quickly. We really liked the aggressive approach of the occupational therapists, and Peter seemed to respond to it well. We got lots of therapy ideas to add to our home repertoire.

The doctors and therapists complimented the family's care of Peter. They felt the progress he had made indicated of a lot of attention and hard work at home. (This, after all, ranked as the most strenuous homeschool "unit study" we'd ever done.)

And they all said, "He's in there, trying to get out."

On Facebook:

November 26, 2010: Looking at What is Unseen; A Message from Mom Friday I returned home from the hospital, where I had been on "Pete duty" for two days. I walked into the house to find the mail on the dining table. There were two cards that had come that day, one from a dear friend in Pennsylvania and one from a dear friend in California. Both had written their cards personally to me. Neither has ever met the other. Both had calligraphed Scripture verses inside their cards. Both "happened" to choose:

"So we do not lose heart. Though our outer nature is wasting away, our inner nature is being renewed day by day. For this slight momentary affliction is preparing for us an eternal weight of glory beyond all

comparison, as we look not to the things that are seen but to the things that are unseen. For the things that are seen are transient, but the things that are unseen are eternal." 2 Corinthians 4:16-18

One of these friends encouraged me in the thought that although Peter's life may appear to be "on hold" right now, God is still working in him, renewing his inner nature. The Holy Spirit is not hindered by comas. This truth lifted my spirits because now that Peter seems more aware of his surroundings, there are times he looks down or discouraged. That my friend is praying for his sanctification to be unhindered, according to the Lord's promise to the believer undergoing affliction, comforts me greatly.

The other friend included in her note her desire that our family time over Thanksgiving might be richer, more meaningful, and more precious than ever. This struck my heart, because my son Peter has always enjoyed time with family so much. So often over the years, I've heard him say following a busy week: "Can we just spend tonight at home as a family?" Peter always felt and appreciated the warmth and security of being close as a family.

Yes, as enjoyable as family fellowship is, in God's scheme of things it is only temporal or transient because it falls into the category of "what is seen." The close fellowship our family has enjoyed over the years in peaceful surroundings is now interrupted somewhat by the jarring nature of Pete's injury. But this close fellowship, after all, is only a picture, albeit a beautiful one, of the real thing, which cannot be disrupted for eternity. How wonderful must the real thing be, if as Peter indicated, the "foretaste" gives so much satisfaction?

Chapter 10

I challenge you young moms and dads to make your home a place of warmth and togetherness and security. Give up whatever it costs you to accomplish it. Make it your priority to show your children a marriage that is like the relationship between Christ and us, and to give them a family that inspires holiness accompanied by an unconditional and effectively working love. It will help sustain you in times of disaster when many worldly families fly apart, and it will draw your children to the beauty of the Lord, to what is unseen and eternal.

Selah

December 6, 2010: Update
Peter is still at Baylor and is about to finish his stay there after his ankle surgery nearly a month ago. Right now the plan is for Pete to come home on Friday, but we are still praying that he will progress to the next level of consciousness before that so that he can stay and undergo formal rehab. The neuropsychologist has told us that they're seeing a wider breadth of responses from Peter, but the responses aren't consistent enough. Overall though, Pete seems to be slowly becoming more aware.

Today they are taking Peter's leg casts off and fitting him for new braces. Earlier this week they also fit Peter for a new mouth guard, which will help protect his teeth from his frequent grinding.

Here are the things that you can pray for:

1. *Pray that Peter's language will be restored. This is something we have been praying for a lot recently, not only so that he will be able to understand us when we talk to him, but so that someday he will be able to talk to us again.*

2. Pray that God would use the people who are helping Peter to encourage him. There are days when Peter looks really discouraged and frustrated that he can't communicate with us. Pray that God would give him comfort and strengthen his faith.

For the family,
Hope

Three days before time for Peter to come home, our hopes rose. He had his best day thus far. He was very alert for the therapists, and while he was still not ready for rehab, he seemed so close.

The neuropsychologist got Pete to look in different directions, and sometimes Peter even moved his head. The doctor also got Peter to wiggle his toes. After his therapy session with Pete, the doctor told Doug to take this opportunity, while Pete was so alert, to tell him everything that is going on in our lives. The speech therapist later put a cap over Peter's trach to allow air to flow through his throat and over his vocal cords. He tolerated it very well, but made no effort to speak.

The day before Peter left Baylor, the new head of the Baylor trauma unit (Dr. Carrington had retired just after Peter's first stay) came in and spoke bluntly with us.

"Now I can't make you any promises," she said. "But here's what I can tell you. Peter is definitely not vegetative. If he were, I could be very sure about his prognosis: that he would not recover. But he is definitely in there, aware and watching and listening to his surroundings. That's a state called 'minimally conscious.'"

She went on. "And I can tell you that this rehab hospital has treated hundreds of minimally conscious people and most come

Chapter 10

out of it. In fact, I called up Dr. Carrington, and of all the minimally conscious people who came through her practice, we could only come up with a handful who had not made a recovery, even if not a total recovery."

"I really think he is going to come out of this," she said. "It just may take some time. You may be looking at a year, as severe as his injury was. Just be patient, keep up his therapy, and watch for signs that indicate he has come to a Level 4." She told us just what to look for.

I thanked her. I had been given my assignment.

And so we all kept up our hopes.

Chapter 11

We waste our lives when we do not pray and think and dream and plan and work toward magnifying God in all spheres of life. God created us for this: to live our lives in a way that makes him look more like the greatness and the beauty and the infinite worth that he really is.
—John Piper

A couple of weeks before Christmas, Peter returned from this third hospital stay (his initial seven-week stay in the trauma unit, the first two-week stay at Baylor, and this most recent month-long stay at Baylor). We were excited that he would be home with us for the holidays. And we did more with him and saw more in him.

During the time off, Doug and Andrew took Peter on first trip in the car since the accident in July. They hoisted him into the front seat of our sedan and took him back to Baylor for an outpatient appointment to get his leg casts cut off. During his high school years, Peter had spent a lot of time in the car driving with his dad to Scout meetings, debate competitions, and church, so we hoped that this trip would evoke many memories and thereby stimulate his brain. During the drive, Doug turned on Dennis Prager and

Chapter 11

Michael Medved, their favorite radio talk-show hosts, and told Pete what he thought about the various topics being discussed. For the whole outing, Peter seemed really engaged with his eyes, like he was listening to every word Dad said.

In mid-December, the kids and some others provided Doug and me a getaway to a local bed and breakfast, so we could get some much-needed rest and do some Christmas shopping. The kids spread out the duties of Peter's care between the siblings, a couple of cousins, an aunt, and Gramma. Caleb and Andrew eased Peter down on the mat each day for physical therapy and some exercises. The family enjoyed watching all of the brothers interacting. Over the holidays, they provided some of Pete's best sessions on the mat.

During our Christmas family time, we were able to give Pete more unique brain stimulation. Beth rubbed root beer candy on his lips and tongue, and he seemed to like that. Andrew and Beth played violin duets, while Caleb accompanied on the piano, as Peter, too, had often done. They played all the fiddle music and hymns that the grandparents had loved during Peter's growing-up years.

We also had an extended family Christmas celebration which Peter seemed to really enjoy. After each family gathering, Pete was more engaged and did something we hadn't seen before. At one point, we asked him to look at each of his cousins. As we called out a name, he, with effort, looked intently at each. That was my first reassurance that he not only saw us, but remembered and knew who we were.

And people continued to encourage our hearts to keep going as the New Year dawned.

On Christmas Eve, some old friends we had not seen in some time dropped by with a festive tin of cookies, a card, and a great deal of love. They gave us healing words. They said that praying for Peter this year had taught them the meaning of intercessory prayer.

"For me," the husband related to us, "Peter's injury was a situation where I saw God strengthening my own walk with the Lord and challenging me to pray without ceasing. Never before have I had a situation before where God has just compelled me to pray continually over a period of time." He told us he prayed intensely for Peter every night before he went to bed. His wife echoed his sentiments; she said she woke up "every morning with Peter on her heart. "

Perhaps misled by the cheerful reception we'd managed to give them that night, she then asked me a personal question. "How are you really doing? Is it ever hard?" She had not been the first to wonder how any parent could bear this. "Do you ever cry?" another friend had recently asked.

"Is it ever hard?" Oh, yes.

"Do I ever cry?" Often.

A new post took shape in my mind:

On Facebook:

December 30, 2011: Message from Mom
Over the holidays, our friends and children put together a team to give us five days off. We had been in and out of the hospital since July, and we were tired.

Chapter 11

On the outing, Doug and I took the opportunity to get away and Christmas shop, go to a showing of The Voyage of the Dawn Treader, *and eat out and such. We knew we should be enjoying our time away, but much of our "romantic fling" was spent in grieving. It overtook us and ran away with us, even while we were trying our best to have "fun."*

We spent time in the Fort Worth cultural district, our long-time favorite stomping ground for family outings, since both Andrew and Beth performed many Youth Orchestra concerts in that area. But we inadvertently passed by Steinway Hall, where Caleb and Peter had performed over the years in piano recitals. That was hard. A few nights earlier in December, their long-time friend and teacher had contacted us to tell us that she had dedicated the evening of the Christmas recital to Peter.

Then we accidentally parked at the exact spot where we remember parking when Peter won an award at the Fort Worth Stock Show Art Contest. As the memory thrust itself into our day, it brought hot tears. We had a picnic in the Botanic Gardens, which brought back memories of concerts we had attended there when Peter was a toddler, including how he used to bury his head in Doug's shoulder when the fireworks went off during the 1812 Overture or The Stars and Stripes Forever. Sure, we cried.

And amazingly enough, the other stresses, strains, and sorrows of life didn't politely stand aside while we dealt with Peter's recovery process. Other griefs visited us during our grieving process. Sometimes life can just be burdensome.

I'm so glad the Lord put 2 Corinthians 1 in the Bible—because that "other" Corinthians passage says that he won't give us more than we can bear. In 2 Corinthians 1:8, however, when Paul speaks of God's comfort during affliction, he tells the church that in Asia, he and his companions had experienced a burden "beyond our strength," so that "we despaired of life itself." Even, "we felt that we had received the sentence of death." Apparently he felt it was more than he could bear. Now, this was more like what I had been feeling. Then Paul told what followed: "But that was to make us rely not on ourselves but on God who raises the dead. He delivered us from such a deadly peril, and he will deliver us." Now the part that includes prayer warriors: "You also must help us by prayer, so that many will give thanks on our behalf for the blessing granted us through the prayers of many."

When I read this, it made me so grateful for all the faithful prayers of the Lord's people granted to us this year. You truly can't imagine. Surely your prayers have delivered us from deadly perils of the soul, such as despair and unbelief. No doubt as well, your prayers have battled Satan for the life and recovery of a young man Peter Helms.

So on this last day of our challenging year, I want to extend warmest thanks from all the Helms family for your diligent and fervent prayers. They are availing much. Whatever the Lord makes of Peter's future life, I know the debt he owes will make him belong twice over to the Body of Christ. He will be wholly yours by virtue of the faithful prayers you have offered on his behalf.

Selah

This dear visiting couple who brought a Christmas tin of cookies, was, of course, the hands and the mouth sent to us that

Chapter 11

day by the "Father of mercies and the God of all comfort" to convey his mercy to struggling and sometimes crying pilgrims.

The Father also showed us mercy through our warm memories of Christmases past. It had been our practice for the last twenty-seven years to take time away in early January for a mini-retreat and planning session. We would evaluate the condition of our own souls, do a "marriage review," scrutinize our ministry, and discuss each child's year—all the while looking over each category for strengths that we needed to shore up and weaknesses we needed to refine as we faced the new year. We would pray and ask the Lord to guide us and give us wisdom as we reflected on past and future.

After we reviewed the year with each other, our tradition included meeting individually with each child as a threesome. We would commend them for the virtues we'd seen in them, listen to their own desires and goals for the year ahead, and challenge them in areas requiring some spiritual work. We took pains to do this all in a manner that was thorough but positive. Then the whole family would go out to eat at a favorite restaurant to celebrate the New Year together.

As they grew older, we turned more and more of the evaluation and initiative over to them and just listened, giving feedback and encouragement. It was an art we learned from our desire to give both direction and growing freedom as was fitting for each child. Then, with each child, we would ask the Lord's blessing and direction on his or her coming year.

Of course, in the wee beginnings of 2011, we were enmeshed in home health care and therapy. There was absolutely no time to fit in a project like this annual tradition. We were in survival mode. Planning anything was a joke.

But then one day, as I cleaned out Peter's old closet to make room for more medical supplies, I came across his list of goals for 2009, the year he was sixteen. (We didn't go on our customary retreat in 2010, either, because we were maxed out preparing for Caleb and Hope's January wedding and caring for my ailing mom). I thought his Facebook prayer warriors might appreciate reading what he wrote. And I realized the Lord must mean for us to use Peter's journaled words once again to help us tell of this road of suffering that we were walking him. I am willing to risk that I may "catch it" from Peter one day for posting this, though I'm pretty sure his good-natured acceptance will kick in once the teen-aged proclivity to embarrassment subsides. My comments are in brackets.

On Facebook:

January 7, 2011: Peter's New Year's Goals; A Message from Mom
"Peter Helms' 2009 New Year Resolutions

> "1. Spiritual: allot at least sixty minutes each day for prayer and Bible reading. Set alarm clock at 7:30. Keep a journal.
> "2. Ministry: Keep myself available to help Dad with ministry and evangelism opportunities.
> "3. Family: Ask advice from Andrew and Caleb about Scouts, debate, girls, and life in general. Keep asking Mom and Dad, too.
> "4. Vocation: Start writing a book about the Four Revolutions. [Peter has been fascinated for a long time with the modern revolutionary age, and as a senior, age seventeen, gave a lengthy presentation in a Western Civilization class on the American,

Chapter 11

> French, Russian, and Chinese revolutions, the worldviews behind them, and the effects they produced in each culture].
>
> "5. Church: Keep friends like Nathan and Nathan [his two best buddies] accountable. Cultivate friendships with older people in the church.
> "6. Physical: Go to the RAC [fitness center] with Dad three days a week. Run, lift weights, do basketball, etc. Also do pushups and run every day at home.
> "7. Friends: Build friendships with people in debate.
> "8. Miscellaneous: Achieve the rank of Eagle Scout. Complete three merit badges. Have Eagle project 'mulled over' and discussed with relevant parties by April. [Peter actually completed his Eagle project the day before his accident, and his Scoutmaster and several Scout buddies saw the paperwork through all the proper channels. He was awarded the rank of Eagle in November, 2010, while he was in Baylor].
> "9. Work one hour a day on debate."

Now, Peter would want me to make it clear that he didn't meet all these goals, but we go by the proverb: if you aim for the sky, you may get as high as the lamp post, but aiming for the lamp post will only get you a couple feet off the ground.

"So teach us to number our days that we may get a heart of wisdom." Psalm 90:12

Selah

Around the same time, while rummaging through Peter's closet looking for something else, I stumbled across Peter's Goals for 2006. He was thirteen.

On Facebook:

January 10, 2011: Peter's Thoughts on a Past New Year; A Message from Mom
"I think that some of my highlights of 2005 are:

" . . . I am glad that my parents put me in more classes than usual this year so that I might have trust in them more, as a result. I am glad of the numerous books that God has used to strengthen my [doctrine] and my joy in fearing God—The Joy of Fearing God *by Jerry Bridges and* Don't Waste Your Life *by John Piper. I have become, I think, a little less sensitive and a little more teachable. The Holy Spirit has taught me that by thinking I know better what's good for me than others who see my character with its vices every day, I prove that 'the heart is deceitful above all things.' Also, I think I may be growing into a better relationship with my siblings by trying to be benevolent in all things no matter what they do or how hurt I feel. I think this growth was triggered specifically by a conversation I had with Mom months ago about having a Christ-like attitude. . . .*

"Some defeats of 2005 are . . . I have neglected to be on the watch many times. I have done things that I would not want to be exposed on Judgment Day. I need to have a reinforcement of the fact that God sees all, but more than that, I hope I will shun evil and desire to glorify God in what I say, do, and think, even if I am alone. . . .

Chapter 11

"Sometimes I don't take pleasure in spiritual subjects and do not wish to partake in them. I think a product of this attitude is being too silly and trying to avoid being serious at the right times. . . . I hope that by the Spirit's work in me, I can avoid this tendency and be diligent and eager in sharing spiritual thoughts with believers and nonbelievers.

"The chief end of man is to glorify God and enjoy him forever. This coming year, by God's grace, I hope that I can strive with zeal and vigor to proclaim God's worthiness and show my joy in him to the world. I hope I can learn more about his sovereignty and love so that I will pour forth in praise to the Lord Jesus. I hope that I will this year, glorify God in everything and in every way, and avoid any excuses for not glorifying God. . . .

"1. I hope I can improve and strengthen my prayer life. I resolve not to make prayer something I only do on evenings or at church. I also resolve to pray earnestly and without holding anything back. As an overshadow or summary, I resolve to pray to God, and not to ceremony or to myself.

"2. . . . I hope I can have an earnest and serious demeanor when I pray and read my Bible. Time-wise, I hope I can be diligent enough in my reading of the Bible to finish it all by the end of 2006. But more importantly, I hope that the Holy Spirit will use what I read to strengthen me spiritually.

"3. I also resolve to be a minister spiritually to everyone I come into contact with. With the body of believers, I hope I can be diligent in encouraging them spiritually, even if they do not return it. With nonbelievers, I hope I can minister to them with compassion and boldness, not telling them what they want to hear, or what I feel I have the courage to say, but rather what the Bible says. . . .

"4. Vices to kill: Pride — confess with humility to God specific instances of pride, rather than just saying 'Please forgive me for all the pride I exhibited today.' Also, make it a practice to ask forgiveness of the fellow men that I offended by my proud attitudes.

Anger — consider that if God had justly carried out his righteousness anger against mankind, I would languish in Hell. Seek to emulate God's mercy. Also, there is an infinitely greater distance between Christ and sinners than between me and the person that has wronged me.

"5. Virtues to strengthen: Obedience to parents — realize that they know more than I do and that they love me. Also, realize that as I am obeying them, I am obeying God. Exodus 20. Holiness — realize that no thought is neutral. Either it is glorifying to God or dishonoring to him. Strive to have praiseworthy and true thoughts. Destroy anything in me that would promote unholiness. Meekness — consider Christ's meek example in suffering for sinners. Also, James 3:17 says that meekness is a characteristic of wisdom.

"Resolved to:
- Read the Bible through with humbleness and a pure attitude.
- Strive to bring specific sins into light and to destroy them.
- Make it a regular practice to talk to my peers about spiritual things. Lead, don't just follow.
- Keep fellow believers accountable. Confront when I have to. Also, listen when they confront me.
- Minister to believers of all ages. Don't hold back if they are a lot different than me. Galatians 3:28.
- If possible, continue 'Christ in the Classics' sculpture series.

Chapter 11

- *Maintain friendships with Joe, Nathan, and Reuben, and develop good friendships with the Hughes boys. Don't close doors to other friendships just because I have good ones right now.*
- *Write edifying emails to brothers during 2006 [Andrew and Caleb were both at college in Tennessee that year].*
- *Improve in friendliness, etiquette and good 'hostmanship.'"*

Sometime in the late fall, we had been contacted by a Virginia couple whose seventeen-year-old son had come across the PRAY FOR PETER HELMS Facebook group as a result of their affiliation with the national homeschool speech and debate organization that Pete was also part of. They offered to give our whole family a week off from Peter's care. The husband is an anesthesiologist, and the wife had been an occupational therapist before she took time out to rear and homeschool their six children. So they were perfectly outfitted to care for Peter.

We prayed and conversed with them by phone and were eventually inclined to take them up on their offer. We agreed on a date in early January, when they were already planning to pack up all their belongings in Virginia and move to Washington, where he had been appointed to a new position on a military base.

We had never actually laid eyes on them before they showed up at our front door.

On their arrival, it seemed as if we had known them all along; they definitely bore the "family resemblance" (to Christ, that is). So we felt completely confident in their love, their abilities, and their care of our son while we spent some good time together as a family and Doug put in some extra time on pastoral duties.

On Facebook:

January 21, 2011
Last week, we said good-bye to some new, near, and dear friends who were driving across the country and wanted to stop by on their way through Texas and give us five days of respite care. The entire family was refreshed by the break.

Peter continues to make small improvements—in holding up his head longer, in recognition of objects and family members, in cooperating with our efforts to strengthen his muscles during mat sessions, and so on.

Prayer requests:

1. *That we will have wisdom, as we care for him at home, to catch anything that needs a doctor's attention.*
2. *That we will be patient with the back-and-forth progress of a brain injury. One doctor told us that recovery from a brain injury was like a graph of the stock market—a lot of ups and downs, highs and lows, but overall trending upward.*
3. *That the Lord will provide a few medical people to help us with his care when he is at home. Also, that the Lord will provide other needed help through the Body of Christ.*

Selah

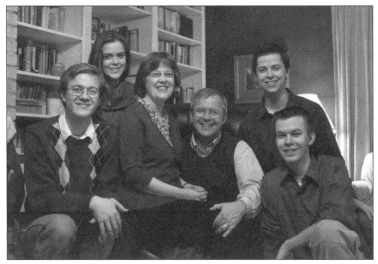

The Helms Family: Christmas 2009

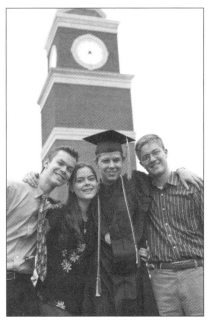

Andrew, Caleb, Beth and Peter: Caleb's graduation from Union University 2009

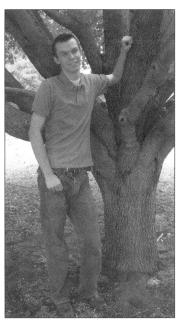

Peter's high school senior picture: May, 2010

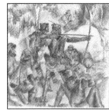

Inset: Colored pencil drawing of Robin Hood and his merry men, age 15

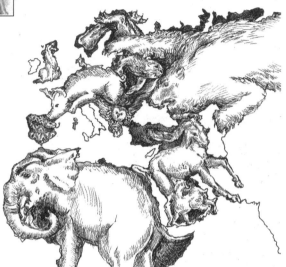

Pen and ink of a doodle on countries and continents, age 16

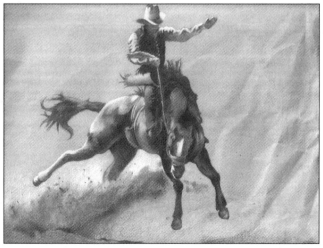

Grand Prize at the Fort Worth Stock Show art contest, age 11

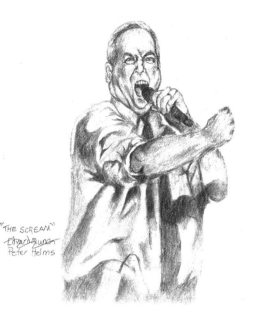

Spoof on democratic presidential candidate Howard Dean, age 14

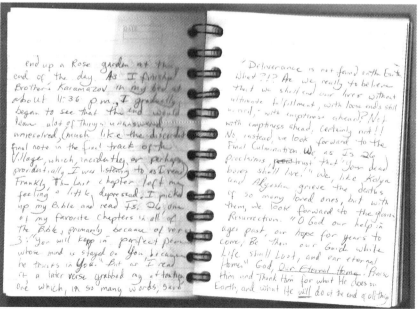

Entry from Peter's journal on his 16th birthday, August 11, 2008

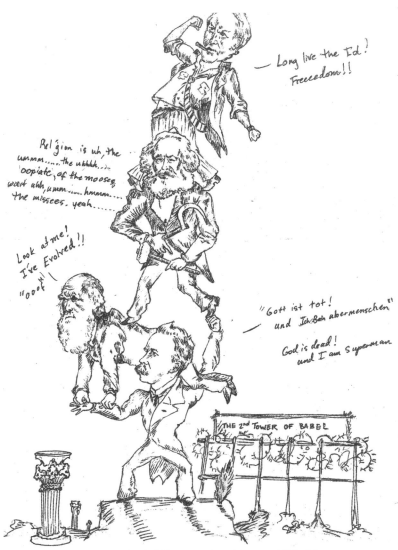

Pen and ink "The American Tower of Babel,"
Pete's critique of Freud, Marx, Nietzsche, and Darwin, age 17

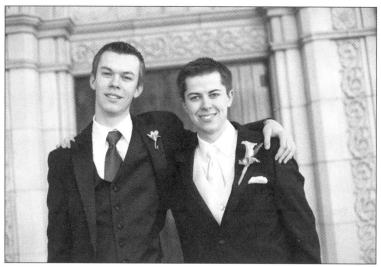

Peter and Caleb at Caleb's wedding: January 2010

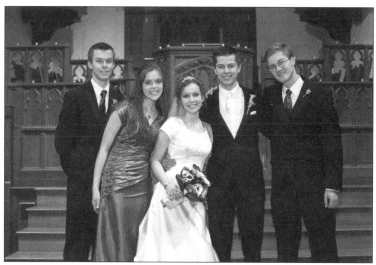

The Helms siblings and their new sister-in-law, Hope, 2010

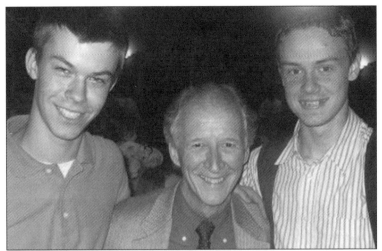

Peter and a friend with John Piper

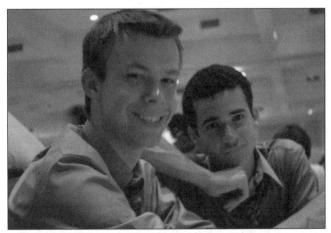

Peter and a friend in speech and debate, senior year, 2010

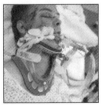

Peter in ICU, after his accident, July 29, 2010

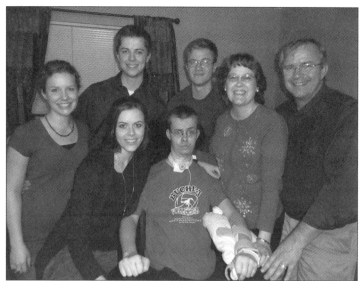

The Helms family, Christmas 2010

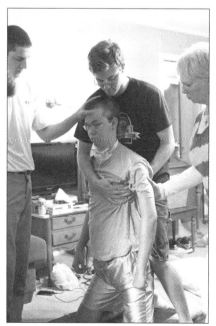

Andrew heading up mat session, 2011

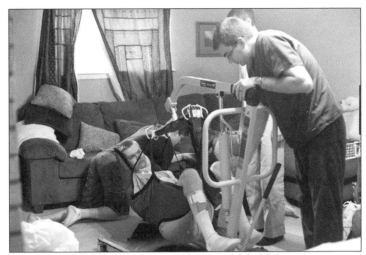

Mat session using the Hoyer lift, 2011

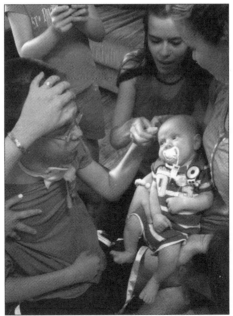

Nephew Winston (born May, 2012)
being employed for "baby" therapy
during mat session

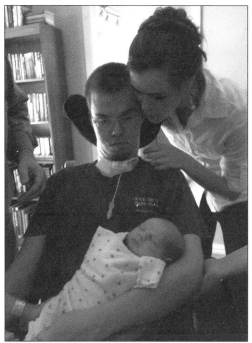
Beth and Peter and Winston, Spring 2012

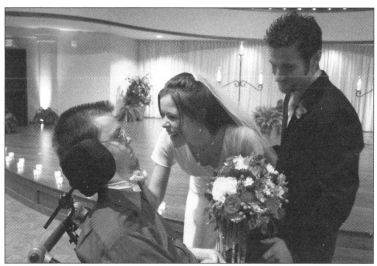
With Beth and Joshua at their wedding, June, 2012

Chapter 12

For those who fight for it life has a flavor the sheltered will never know.
— Theodore Roosevelt

In the early days of 2011 we struggled to settle into our new "normal." This included grieving for the loss of our beloved son as we had known him, assuming the care of a totally dependent invalid on a trach, doing four to six hours of therapy a day for a TBI patient—a combination of tasks which absorbed our total concentration. We had learned to suction a trach, to put a meal through a feeding tube, to crush ten pills at a time, and to administer breathing treatments. We had learned to stay awake all night and listen for signals from Pete that he needed our help. We had learned to turn him every two hours and to give bed baths. We had learned passive range-of-motion exercises and upper airway anatomy for effective speech therapy. And we had learned how to place objects in his hands and cognitively challenge him to move the object we named.

That month we decided we needed to reintroduce Peter to as many of his past social circles as we could. We took Peter to church for "Sanctity of Life" Sunday late in January. Doug swung him

Chapter 12

up into our aging suburban using the one-man lift he'd learned at Baylor. I packed up an old cooler with his supplies. It took two of us to get his one hundred-pound wheelchair folded into the back of the car. The effort it took for Andrew, Doug, and me to prepare Pete for the outing effectively squelched any nervousness we might have been tempted to feel. By the time we backed cautiously from the driveway, we were all sweating with the exertion, no energy left for anticipating what could go wrong.

It was his first time back at our little church since his accident six months earlier. Everyone greeted him warmly, and he appeared to enjoy being there.

Doug had first taken this pastorate almost twelve years earlier, when Peter was six, so Pete had grown up taking pages of sermon notes with "Bro. Dad" listed at the top as the speaker. Surely, being back at Rock Creek would spur memories for Peter.

Several people had not seen him since his accident, and, as might be expected in a small church after half a year, there were new faces Pete had never seen before. I wondered how people would see him: Peter as our good-natured and strapping 6'4" young man, or Peter as invalid. Would people be able to look beyond the wheelchair to see the dignity and value of my son's precious life? (Hopefully a reasonable question to ask on pro-life Sunday!) Pete still could not speak or control his muscles or always focus his eyes on the person speaking to him. Would that keep people from seeing him as we have known him for eighteen years: winsome, humble, intelligent, and so much more?

We belong to a hardy church family that responded to Peter and his needs with dignity and love. The mother of one of Peter's best friends told him, "Little brother, I miss having you play basketball in my driveway."

Another elderly woman called him "my Peter" and assured him of her frequent prayers. Men shook hands with him and filled him in on the news of their own lives.

We agreed afterward that the outing had been a success. Even as an invalid — *especially* as an invalid — Peter would need the support of his church family. We would all, as a church family, have a front-lines role in the battle for the dignity of human life. And these dear people would form a big part of the support team that made it possible for us to care for Peter in our home. A new post took form:

On Facebook:

January 31, 2011: Sanctity-of-Life Message from Mom
For those who might be unfamiliar with this phrase — sanctity of life — I use it to describe the implications of God having made man in his own image, uniquely fashioned for fellowship with him. (On this basis, for example, the Lord prohibits murder in the Ten Commandments.) Thus, all human beings, regardless of their ability or disability, race, age, gender, or social class, have been created in God's image and are to be treated as persons of equal worth and inviolable dignity. Human life is precious. We believe that this principle, practically applied, makes abortion, euthanasia, and suicide offenses against God and man.

Doug says that what we are doing at home with Peter makes a strong sanctity-of-life statement. Peter and Doug so often in the past sat across the table from each other, eating cheeseburgers together in joy and fellowship, and though we now feed Peter through a stomach tube, Doug says that if we do it with love and eagerness, we give Satan's cause a black eye. And every time we get up and turn Peter in the night, and do it with joy, we proclaim how precious Peter's life is. And every time we give him a "range-of-motion" patiently and thoroughly, we take ground for the Lord's kingdom. There are spiritual beings who watch us in the privacy of our home. The angels look on and rejoice when they see us treating Peter's life as sacred. Ephesians 3 tells us that the wisdom of God is made known to the rulers and authorities in the heavenly places through Christ's church and what his people do.

So many of you have those in your own lives who are weak and cannot speak for themselves: from the unborn to the elderly. Surely, the way we treat these, who are all around us, reveals our hearts. Each person has potential and giftedness and value and a story. Do we treat them with the dignity due God's image-bearers, seeing all the creative sides to their unique personalities, treating them as individuals worthy of getting to know? When we do, we shout to the world, seen and unseen, the sanctity of the lives God has entrusted to us.

I have used this Facebook group to celebrate my son's life. May it inspire everyone to take pleasure in the worth of all those individuals God has placed within your own sphere.

"The thief comes only to steal, kill and destroy. I have come that they might have life, and have it more abundantly." John 10:10

Selah

February 9, 2011

Thank you for sharing. Your family and your faith are an encouragement to my soul. I am spurred on to love Jesus more, to seek joy in all things. You all are incarnating Christ beautifully. We pray for you often here.

Chelsea

Through the months of January, February, March, and April, Peter progressed slowly, but well. He continued to make small improvements during his therapy sessions on the floor mat. Even though we still totally assisted him, his muscles grew stronger and he could bear some of his own weight from a kneeling or crawling position. His body began to assume the exercise positions more naturally, instead of us having to hold his limbs in place. We would also pull his arms forward, away from the back support of the wheelchair, hoping his core muscles would firm up. As they did, he became able to hold his head up for several seconds at a time.

Because Pete's neck muscles were stronger, he did better with his capping trials (during which we partially capped his trach so he had to breathe through his nose). There were days he could breathe effortlessly for two or three hours at a time.

We took him in the car to church every couple of weeks, Andrew and Doug teaming up to do the "one man" lift. As far as we could tell, Pete seemed to enjoy it. Sometimes the stimulation wore him out so much that on Mondays and Tuesdays, he wouldn't do much but sleep. So we didn't take him every week.

Pete also continued to look at people on command. He still lacked consistency, but occasionally, when he seemed really alert, we asked him to look at specific people and he would move his

Chapter 12

eyes and his head to accomplish it. Sometimes, we made it more challenging for him, asking him to "Look at Nathan's big brother," or "Look at the girl who calls you 'Chubs,'" or "Look at the guy who's courting Beth." On his best days, he could nail a whole string of correct responses to these simple commands. It was probably one of the most encouraging things we saw him do because it let us know that he had memory and language recognition and cognitive associations.

We had to be patient in between such responsive times, since he would sometimes drift off again for days. But when he did peg ten or twelve answers in a row, it really cheered us. He also gained awareness of what was going on in the next room. He would occasionally glance over when he heard activity, whereas, earlier, he was only aware of us when we were a few feet from him.

Peter also seemed to be rediscovering that he had a mouth. His jaws had stayed clenched shut for months, but now he began to open his mouth sometimes to make chewing or speaking motions. We'd tell him, "Come on, Peter, keep at it, we want to feed you a cheeseburger soon," and "Come on, Pete, say something," as it looked so much at times as if he wanted to speak. Whenever Beth entered the room to do speech therapy with him, his face lit up and we were sure he would speak to her at any moment.

On Facebook:

February 18, 2011
Here are the things you can pray for:

1. *Pray for Peter's spiritual and emotional encouragement.*

2. Andrew has been by his little brother's side on this whole road of suffering. Andrew flew down from Indiana on the day Peter had his accident (when we didn't know whether or not he would live), and has rarely left Peter's bedside since. As he had just completed his first year as a PhD student in philosophy at Notre Dame, he asked for, and was graciously given, a year's personal leave of absence without losing his position there. Though the family, and so much of the extended family have pitched in to help with Peter's care, Andrew is the one who does not live in this area. We are asking the Lord to let Andrew see some of the fruit of his many hours of vigil and labor with Peter before he resumes his scholastic life. Andrew has been a witness to so many of the medical people we've rubbed shoulders with over the past months. Many of them have marveled at the sacrificial investment he has given to his brother. He just replies to them, "Well, he's my brother, and I love him," as if to say, "What else would I have done?"
3. Pray that Peter would begin regaining his speech. This would be a great thing for Andrew to see before he leaves.

For the family,
Hope

March 3, 2011: Thank You
Thanks to all of you who posted on Peter's group wall, sent him messages and notes after my request. It blessed us to read all the encouragements to him, and they continually lifted our spirits, as we trust they did for him. We received messages in every possible form of communication, and everyone's words have given us grace to keep going. May the Lord richly

Chapter 12

bless all of you for coming alongside Pete on this road of suffering and recovery.

Hope

One of the heart-breaking things about Peter's injury was the effect it had on other people. Our youngest son was engaging and friendly and a favorite in our circles. Now, when we were in public, people stared, or tried not to. Even people who knew Peter before his accident sometimes didn't know what to say to him, or they spoke to him much differently than they had before. Some avoided him altogether. And although the children of our church had always hung on him and begged him to come outside and play with them, now children were very shy around Peter. Some kids were scared of him. Medical people, though well-intentioned and helpful, treated him much differently as a patient than they would have had he been the Peter we had previously known and loved. A severe brain injury that renders a person unable to communicate is the worst sort of disability for social acceptability.

March 15, 2011: At Home in the Body; A Message from Mom
Now that we have had Peter out more with other people, there have been a couple of times when it's been hard on someone to see him in his current condition. One or two people have said, "That's not Peter," as if his limitations somehow change who he is. I understand this struggle. The topic has fostered many questions and discussions in our own home. Frankly, it has really helped me to share a home with a philosopher/theologian son

(Andrew) and a pastor/theologian husband. Their words give me sound perspective.

The Christian view confronts head-on this temptation to focus too much on Peter's brain. Our culture's worldview says that our personhood is equal to our brain. That's because materialism holds that we are only physical beings, that we are nothing more than what can be seen or touched.

The Christian view, on the other hand, is that each of us has a soul that will never die. This soul we each have is the essence of who we are. Our souls equal our personhood. Our bodies are only our habitation, like a tent, while we live on this earth. Our bodies certainly are a wondrous gift with which God graced us so that we can learn about and serve him. Yet, they are only a vehicle for the real "us."

So Peter's soul—who he is—has not changed. His brain is part of his tent. His brain is a tool that his soul uses, and the tool has been hurt. He is still the same Peter that we have always known and not anyone "different."

Since Peter is still essentially the same, we focus on his soul and not his brain. He needs our spiritual encouragement, our moral support. We want to support him on this road of suffering he has been called to walk. He's still our little brother.

"For we know that if the tent, which is our earthly home is destroyed, we have a building from God, a house not made with hands, eternal in the heavens. For in this tent we groan, longing to put on our heavenly dwelling . . . . For while we are still in this tent, we groan, being burdened—not that we would be unclothed, but that we would be further *clothed, so that what is mortal may be swallowed up by life. He who has prepared us for this very thing is God, who has given us the Spirit as a guarantee.*

"So we are always of good courage. We know that while we are at home in the body we are away from the Lord . . . . (W)e would rather be away from the body and at home with the Lord. So whether we are at home or away, we make it our aim to please him." 2 Corinthians 5:1-9

Selah

In March, we were informed that Peter's old debate club planned to hold a tournament in his honor as a fundraiser for him. We were so thankful for those who contributed their time, energy, and resources to pulling off the event, and the efforts to lower their costs so that the contribution to Peter's medical needs could be maximized. Doug, Andrew, and I all attended portions of the event. Many who knew Peter approached us with kind and encouraging words. Their caring and generous and prayerful spirits lifted our hearts. We met Tim Laitinen, a young Christian man who edited a Christian magazine for singles. Tim convinced Andrew to meet him for coffee and an interview. Then he published an article about how God's gift of singleness to Andrew had allowed him the freedom to minister wholeheartedly to his younger brother:

Solo Zone: Flexibility in a Crisis
By Tim Laitinen
Imagine getting that phone call: a loved one has been involved in a horrible traffic accident in another state.

Can you freeze-frame your life at that moment, putting everything else on hold to jump on a plane to be at your loved one's hospital bedside?

Of course, many people can't. But Andrew Helms could. A single doctoral student at Indiana's University of Notre Dame, Helms rushed to consult with his advisors, and then scrambled to the airport for a flight home to Texas.

Granted, working on a doctorate doesn't require the same type of on-site commitment and responsibility as being professionally employed. But neither can graduate studies be easily maintained when you're fraught with the relentless urgency of having a loved one undergo multiple surgeries, in different hospitals, by various specialists, with progress measured in barely discernable increments—all of which awaited Andrew and his family as his brother's long road to recovery began that summer day last year.

Brother, Can You Spare the Time?

At eighteen years old, Peter is Andrew's youngest brother, with two other siblings in the middle. Being the oldest has always given Andrew a tendency to play the role of protector for his brothers and sister, despite what he describes as "a healthy mixture of camaraderie and rivalry" between them.

"They are specially placed in my life for me to practice the discipline of brotherly love," Andrew unabashedly reasons. "It's easier to see how much they need my love when they are in trouble."

For the first few hours after that initial, crisis phone call, nobody really knew if Peter would survive. His small car had been broadsided by a

Chapter 12

full-sized pickup truck at full speed, and witnesses to the crash assumed the worst until paramedics arrived and managed to find a pulse. They rushed Peter by helicopter to a Fort Worth trauma center, where he was quickly assessed to have facial puncture wounds and broken bones, as well as severe bleeding in his brain.

Surgeons were able to drill a hole in Peter's skull to relieve some of the pressure on his brain, and they believed his spinal cord had been spared serious injury. And the Lord spared his life.

But little else.

Today, after ten months and several surgeries, Peter remains in a minimally conscious state, unable to communicate or voluntarily move his body except for slight twitches and eye movements. Although the progress that has taken place has been a blessing, that progress has been disappointingly slow in coming. Yet family members have rallied around, joined by congregants from their church and friends around their Fort Worth community who have supported the family in ways we never realize we need until such a crisis.

Most days, everyone's time is spent maintaining a steady regimen of physical therapy so Peter's limbs retain a range of motion and flexibility. Doctors remain hopeful about his prognosis, but he's yet to reach the point where he's eligible for intensive rehabilitation. So the family soldiers on with Peter at home, where his hospital bed has commandeered their living room, and everyone's routine now centers around his care.

Lessons of Faith and Purpose

The emotional, physical, and even spiritual toll on Peter's family and friends has been immense, but at the same time, profoundly faith-building. As a doctoral philosophy student, Andrew has developed a keen awareness of how his own relationship with Christ has flourished during what could be a season of despondency.

"During the hardest moments, in the midst of deep grief and fear for Peter and all the things that he seems to have lost, God has sustained and comforted me with this thought: All those things... are gifts from Christ. Everything beautiful and praiseworthy in Peter is a direct reflection of Christ's beauty and praiseworthiness. Therefore, nothing is really lost; instead, we're being directed to look up from the broken image, back to the Person who formed it to resemble himself, and who really possesses those good things by right."

Of all the truths God may be revealing about himself by allowing Peter's present condition, Andrew sees a particular relevance for all saints who suffer.

"In the present difficult circumstances, Peter has been given the great gift of reflecting and identifying with Christ in his humiliation and suffering. If that's the case, then, because of his unity with Christ, Peter will be exalted and restored someday. So, this injury is actually a gift straight from the hand of a gracious God who plans for Peter to be holy... rather than a gifted artist or an intellectual genius."

Andrew also can't escape less complex reminders about the purposes of community in faith.

"God's been helping me see that for us Christians, human relationships are the training ground for, and entry into, close communion with himself. The presence of other people in our lives calls for us to develop deep habits of sacrifice and self-giving. We have to learn humility by sacrificing our desires to the good of others, as bearers of the image of God."

This Present Present of Singlehood

This, in a way, helps to explain why Andrew's singleness has been an odd sort of blessing. His professors at Notre Dame graciously offered him a leave of absence for a year to help with his brother's recovery. So Andrew simply stayed in Texas after flying down the day of Peter's accident, relieved to be able to support his family without competing responsibilities.

"Given Peter's accident, I am grateful for my current state of singleness," Andrew acknowledges. *"Being unmarried has made it much easier than it would have been for me to give my time and effort towards his care and rehabilitation. . . . I had this freedom to change my location and devote my time to helping my brother for a year. I don't know what I would have done in other circumstances.*

"As a Christian who is unmarried, I am trying to use the free time that I have — that would have been used up caring for a wife and a family — in service to Christ and his church. This year, that means serving my brother in his time of need."

Granted, a one-year hiatus during his pursuit of a doctorate won't be catastrophic to Andrew's career. It's even been educational in itself.

"It has changed me as a person: made me more grateful, more confident, more loving, less afraid of what people think of me," he reflects.

As his hiatus from Notre Dame starts winding down, and as his brother's condition continues to stabilize, Andrew has begun looking towards the future once more. And although singlehood has been a unique advantage so far, he's willing to, shall we say, broaden his relationship horizons.

"I hope that God's plan for me involves marriage in the near future," he admits. "At the same time, I am not waiting on marriage to make me happy or give me purpose in life. I already have those things in Christ."

In spite of the slow progress back home, Pete made a small breakthrough during a session on the floor mat. We had regularly instructed him to look at specific people. Sometimes he could; sometimes he couldn't. One day I decided to push the limits of what he had done so far.

First I asked him to look at Beth, which he did. Then Beth and I proceeded to talk in a regular tone about miscellaneous things. After about two minutes, I calmly asked Peter to look at Andrew (who was on Pete's other side), and he did so immediately and deliberately. This was really encouraging to us because it meant that Peter could filter out personal commands from general chit chat, a great feat for a TBI patient because they often can't focus enough to respond in the midst of distractions or multiple stimulations.

Also at this time, we began to remodel our house to better accommodate Peter's needs and ours. He needed more privacy. We needed our living room to be available once again for visitors and counseling and a myriad of other pastoral and family uses. We also wanted to designate a specific place where we could organize all the many supplies necessary for Peter's care.

We destroyed a bedroom closet to make a new doorway from that bedroom into the kitchen/dining area. This would become Peter's room, from which he could always overhear the buzz of family activities. We also redid the bathroom to fit Peter's wheelchair into the shower. We eventually installed hardwood floors so that Pete could be wheeled around the house without buckling the carpet and tearing loose its edges. All of this had to be accomplished with minimal dust and debris that might interfere with Peter's trach. The house was decorated for many weeks with tarp tents.

April 17, 2011: Trusted with a Trial? A Message from Mom
Last week Doug traveled to Mexico City to preach at a pastors' conference. As the time got closer for him to leave, my worries ran faster. "What were we thinking?" "Why did we decide for him to do this when so much of Peter's care involves his dad?" "And to Mexico?" I became pretty much a basket case. And I share this, not to be a whiner, but to give me a chance to boast in the Lord, who provided much help the week Doug was gone. Our need gave him many opportunities to display his strength.

People have said to us over these months: "You are so strong," and "The Lord knew he could trust you with a trial like this." I so appreciate the heartfelt goodwill behind these words, yet I want to reveal candidly to everyone that we are not strong, not for a single moment that he is not carrying us. I am, frankly, a weakling.

We have learned through this experience that heavy trials come to all sorts of people, irrespective of their spiritual strength. God doesn't just pick the strong ones. In fact, since we have run in medical circles associated with brain trauma patients, we have discovered that not only is brain injury epidemic in our country, but that it often explodes families into fragments because of the daunting challenges accompanying it. The night nurse we have employed to help with Peter was released from a recent position in which he was nurse to another young man whose parents ended their marriage because of the stress related to their son's injury.

And there are often times when Doug and I feel unequal to the task of walking through this trial. There are times we are weak and exhausted. There are times we feel we can't go another step.

Clearly, we have seen that it is the Lord, and not our own strength, that sustains us, or any believer, through trial. We have never felt our human weakness more keenly. But as well, we have never been more aware of how the Lord keeps his people bearing up under trial. He gives any believer grace for whatever he sends, not based on where we are in our Christian walks. We don't have to be strong beforehand; he gives the strength when the moment of trial is upon us. In fact, it's through the trial that believers understand the depth of our weakness and dependency on our Lord to carry us. Our continual story is how the Lord uses his Word and the hymns and prayers of his people to comfort and compose our hearts.

So let me share with you how God gives us grace: when I am sure my fatigue will keep me in bed till noon, grace comes in the form of a delicious meal that arrives on our doorstep, or in the form of three women who appear at my front door, ready to clean my house for the umpteenth time this year. When I am sure my health is about to break down, grace comes in the form of green juice (yes, I am a health food freak) that is left on our front porch bench from sisters trying to keep me healthy. Recently, when I was especially discouraged, strength came in the form of a package in the mail, arriving from friends in Pennsylvania. Inside were CDs full of hymn arrangements. Sometimes when I have wondered if my faith would even make it through this trial, I have heard a sermon that bolsters my shaky faith to keep going.

Three weeks ago, grace came by the hand of a young nursing student from Union University (where Peter was scheduled to go), who asked if we would allow her to give us her spring break to help care for Pete. That really gave us a chance to rejuvenate. And in just the past several days I took calls from Christian sisters in California, Texas, and Tennessee who remind my wimpy heart of the truth of God's love and faithfulness and of their faithful prayers for Peter.

Every time we sing together as a family in the evenings, when someone suggests Peter's favorite hymn, I am awestruck at what the Lord put on Peter's heart back when he could talk. Almost every time his turn had come around the previous couple of years, he'd chosen this song:

> *"Jesus, I my cross have taken,*
> *All to leave and follow thee,*
> *Destitute, despised, forsaken,*
> *Thou from hence my all shalt be.*
> *Perish every fond ambition,*
> *All I've sought or hoped or known,*
> *Yet, how rich is my condition:*
> *God and heaven are still my own.*

"Go then earthly fame and treasure;
Come disaster, scorn and pain.
In Thy service pain is pleasure,
With Thy favor, loss is gain.
I have called Thee, 'Abba, Father;'
I have stayed my heart on Thee:
Storms may howl and clouds may gather,
All must work for good to me."

These words must have been foreknown by the Lord as the lyrics that would comfort us every time we choose the song for Peter's turn. When I am sad, they cheer me every time. And we as a family have enjoyed rich times of strengthening around Peter's bed, fellowshipping in the evenings. God gave us this and other hymns to impart his strength to us in our faltering walk. Truly he carries his dear children along.

"But he said to me, 'My grace is sufficient for you, for my power is made perfect in weakness.' Therefore I will boast all the more gladly of my weaknesses, so that the power of Christ may rest upon me. For the sake of Christ, then, I am content with weaknesses, insults, hardships, persecutions, and calamities. For when I am weak, then I am strong." 2 Corinthians 12:9, 10

Selah

Chapter 13

How often have we told our hearers, that our all-sufficient and faithful Lord can and will make good every want and loss! How often have we spoken of the light of his countenance as a full compensation for every suffering, and that trials of this present life are not worthy to be compared with the exceeding abundant and eternal weight of glory to which they are leading! We must not therefore wonder if we are sometimes called to exemplify the power of what we have said, and to show our people that we have not set before them unfelt truths, which we have learnt from books and men only. You are now in a post of honour, and many eyes are upon you. May the Lord enable you to glorify him, and to encourage them, by your exemplary submission to his will.
— John Newton to a fellow pastor

The spring hurried by while Peter's progress lagged. There were few new things to report. His doctors had warned us that Pete may have plateaus in his short-term healing, but that it didn't necessarily indicate a long-term plateau.

Allergy season hit, and Peter grew tired and sluggish. The air quality was poor for normally breathing people, much more for those dependent on trachs. Congestion prevented him from sleeping, which in turn made him less responsive to therapy during the days. In spite of this, he made somewhat steady progress at people recognition, so we expanded our exercises with him to include object and picture recognition.

Pete was not as consistent on object/picture recognition as he had been with people. For instance, we could tell him "Pete look down the hall!" and he might seem confused, but when we said "Pete, look at the refrigerator!" he often nailed it immediately. This had obviously been an intimate object to him in the past.

Peter made some larger motor movements too, but he still didn't have any control over them at this point. We frequently pulled him up to a standing position so he would bear weight on his legs. He could keep his legs straight for a while, but eventually they would buckle.

Pete also moved his mouth more frequently. He began taking food from a spoon, anything with pudding-like consistency. At first he made terrible faces at the taste since he was so unused to tasting. Our speech therapist called this oral aversion, common in stroke or brain-injured patients.

Though his progress seemed infinitesimal, we continued to hope and look for Level 4 on the Rancho Scale (when he would respond consistently to several simple commands). We kept hearing stories of amazing brain injury recoveries that kept us working patiently with Pete, day after day. One friend from church told us of a neurologist nurse who had long cared for a young man who was minimally conscious. After two years, he "woke up" to the next level of consciousness, asked for pizza, and made a recovery.

Throughout Peter's slow spring, we began to face up to Andrew's looming departure for Notre Dame. He would leave behind big shoes, and we had to figure out how to fill them. The Lord provided us with a capable, loving day nurse who learned how to do much of what had been Andrew's responsibilities.

In July, Peter went to a new doctor who had worked with many traumatic brain injury patients over the years. He was very encouraging to us and said he thought that Peter would make a substantial recovery; it would just take time.

There were a few times when Peter seemed to be a little more aware of what was going on around him. During these times, we challenged him with more complicated questions. For example, we began holding up a Bible and a hymnal next to each other and asking, "Which book has *A Mighty Fortress* in it?" and waiting to see if he would find the correct object, rather than saying "Look at the hymnal." We also held up "yes" and "no" cards, and asked him questions like, "Peter, is *Genesis* one of the Gospels?" and "Is *Luke* in the Old Testament?" On days when he was really on his game, he could answer fifteen or twenty of these in a row with 95 percent accuracy. We hoped this would become consistent, indicative of another small step in Peter's recovery process.

As Peter had more success in answering these types of questions, it seemed to that he might have more of a "locked-in syndrome" in which he heard and understood far more than he could respond to. There were definitely times when we felt like Pete evidenced a keen awareness of his situation, such as when we occasionally found him crying.

Hope posted that month's prayer requests with an update:

On Facebook:

. . . . *In other news, we have changed Peter's diet to get him off of the canned liquid food that was full of sugar. For a week Pete seemed to feel pretty bad as he had to detox, but we have seen a lot of good results since then because of the change in diet. We have also finished the bulk of the remodeling that needed to be done in the house! Peter now has his own room right off the kitchen and a wheelchair-accessible shower.*

We have a few big prayer requests right now in addition to the usual ones for strength and patience:

1. *Shortly after Peter's accident, Andrew's back started hurting. Over the last year, as Andrew helped care for Peter, his back became worse and worse. Recently, we found out that Andrew has a herniated disk. He is in a lot of pain, and we need wisdom to know how to help him before he returns to Notre Dame in less than a month.*
2. *Pray that the Lord will provide a wheelchair-accessible van. Dad has been taught a one-man lift to get Peter in and out of a vehicle, but this also strains his back. We think it's now time to explore a better option.*
3. *Pray that we will be able to establish some form of "yes" and "no" communication with Peter. This would be helpful in our care for him on so many levels, and also give Peter a way to express himself.*
4. *Please continue to pray that Peter's secretions would clear up so that he can rest and so that his trachea won't be irritated from the constant hacking.*

Thank you, friends!
Hope

Chapter 13

Dear Hope, Doug, Selah and family,

Thanks for the update — Anita told us about Peter's accident when we queried the comments on her Facebook about a year ago, and it has done us good to see how all of you have responded with God's help through very tough times — not that we would wish this on anyone! So there is at least one family down under praying for you guys. Our two children are now thirty-five and thirty-one, so we are somewhat older, but as a father and mother we can understand some of what you must be going through.

Thanks for your ministry to others through these circumstances,

Stan and Elsa Whitman
Adelaide, Australia

One morning that summer, Doug and I had just returned from a workout. I jumped in the shower, while he lugged our trash containers to the front curb. Gramma and our night nurse were getting Peter ready for the day.

Suddenly Gramma was knocking on our bedroom door, calling frantically for Doug. Pounding next on Andrew's door and her call for him further broke the morning quiet in the hallway. Something was wrong.

I dressed quickly and sped into the hall. Doug, Andrew, and I simultaneously made for Peter's room. We saw him blue and struggling to breathe, his trach in his nurse's hand. Gramma had 911 on the phone. Andrew grabbed the ambubag and began trying to force air down Peter's airway through his mouth. I tried to calm both of them, as well as help nurse to get the trach back in, then the oxygen tube into his trach stoma (the surgical hole in his neck). Peter's eyes were wide and panicked. Doug prayed.

The trach had apparently fallen out during Peter's bath. No one saw it at first under the gauze that covered the area. By the time the nurse noticed, Peter's neck and throat muscles had tensed so tightly as to prevent reinsertion.

Within a few minutes, the ambulance arrived. The EMTs were able to force one of their larger oxygen tubes down Pete's airway, but drew blood as well. Getting him to the hospital was urgent.

The attendants administered a shot of epinephrine during transport. At the hospital, it only took a few minutes to stabilize him and get the trach back in. After a few hours' stay, they sent us home.

We crashed for the rest of the day, totally depleted emotionally and physically. I worried that the oxygen deprivation might set Pete back, but the doctors assured us that it would not. Rosemary brought us a rotisserie chicken and hummus. We ate practically lying down on the couch and went to bed as soon as the night nurse showed back up.

The next day, something surprising happened. Peter was more awake. That afternoon he responded successfully to more questions than ever before. For weeks after that scare, he was more alert and aware of his surroundings. We had no way of knowing whether or not this was caused by the shock from the traumatic experience. Regardless, it was nice to see him more alert, even though it was just a slight difference.

So we saw Peter make some small improvements. For instance, sometimes we tried to spoon feed him during speech therapy, and there were occasions when he took up to five small bites of apple sauce in his mouth and swallowed it willingly. Other times,

Chapter 13

Peter moved his head away from the spoon. So it seemed as if he was exercising his will and/or was really agitated by the spoon-feeding—all signs that he could be coming closer to another level of consciousness.

Pete also made progress towards getting weaned off of his trach. We used the speech valve on the trach for several hours each day, forcing him to breathe through his throat. This was satisfying because occasionally we heard Peter groan or grunt due to the airflow over his vocal chords. It really made us look forward to hearing him talk again.

Though we had all thrown our collective energy into arousing the dormant functions of Peter's brain, his progress had been excruciatingly minimal. And I found that when the one-year anniversary of his accident loomed on our calendar, it took a lot of spiritual work to get past it. We determined to keep a positive outlook, still making room for the Lord to bring Peter back to us, no matter what he chose to do in the long run. So we remained undaunted in our efforts, even as we prepared for Andrew to head back to school.

On Facebook:

July 19, 2011: The One Year Mark; A Message from Mom
A year has gone by. One year ago next Thursday, Peter drove to do a morning's yard work for a widow in our church. He was earning a little pocket money for college expenses. Doug and I went to work out at the fitness center; we would see him later in the day. Instead, we got a call from the hospital telling us that our son had barely lived through a horrific car wreck and might not make it through the day.

Now he is in our home. He and his brother Andrew, both history buffs, once tried to stump each other on hard questions: "Who was the French king who went on the fourth Crusade? Which Roman Emperor was a Stoic?" Now, Andrew shows Peter flash cards, hoping he remembers what a cat and a horse and a duck are.

Last year, Peter was eager to spread his wings and live as a young man, managing his own stuff and schedule at school. Now we dress him and feed him every day.

Last year, he was looking forward to sharpening his debate skills on the college debate team, for which, though an incoming freshman, he had earned a varsity scholarship. Today, we pray to hear him speak again.

So day after day, we continue therapy. We try to do one or more hours each of speech therapy, physical and occupational therapy, and cognitive therapy every day, for a total of four to six hours daily, depending on how much sleep he needs. We continue to see small improvements.

You know, the Christian religion, contrary to what many believe, does not fit into that great American ideal of pragmatism. We got that from Ben Franklin, not Christ. We don't follow Christ because "he works" to solve all our problems. We don't trade in our obedience for present-day rewards. We get this notion that if we can just pray with a certain amount of faith, obey all the "Christian" rules, or live by certain "principles," we are guaranteed the Lord's blessings in tangible, earthly manifestations and the timing we think best.

But this is not about "what works." In fact, the Bible is pretty much a story of believers not getting earthly rewards for their following of Christ.

Chapter 13

See Moses, Joseph for years of his life, Isaiah, Jeremiah, Baruch, Paul, Peter, and many other first-century disciples. These people suffered great hardships throughout their lives, some without relief, even while doing what God had given them to do. The message is much more than pragmatism preaches. In truth: you do what's right and leave the results to God.

That ethic guides how we approach Peter. So Doug says that no matter how much recovery Peter ever attains, he would still do mat session daily. We would still keep him beside us and talk to him and read Scripture to him and play Mozart and Rachmaninoff for him and exercise his hands with his basketball. I guess you could call it our version of Martin Luther's idea that if he knew that the world were coming to an end tomorrow, he would still plant a tree today. We do it because he is our son and it is right for us to do this for him, not contingent on any way Peter can pay us back in the future for our investment. Nothing that we do that is beautiful and right and obedient for Christ can ever be wasted.

"Duty is ours; results are God's," claimed an obscure, but dedicated, early American public servant. The tricky part is to do our duty by Peter in the midst of great grief, keeping hopeful spirits upbeat, even while we miss fellowshipping with him so much. As Andrew says, we can never let our sadness drive us away from Peter. Rather, in our sadness, we move towards him and keep loving him. For that, we are daily dependent on the Lord's grace.

Next week, Andrew will return to Notre Dame to pick the academic thread of his life back up and resume the pursuit of his professional calling. He has been a full partner with his parents in this struggle; we have worked together daily to keep each other encouraged in the truth and to comfort each other with the Corinthians comfort of the Lord (2 Corinthians 1). I tremble in my boots over this, though Doug daily reminds me to put my trust in God. We lose not just a hard worker, but a dear and precious friend-in-arms with his absence. What has Andrew received for his labor? From an earthly perspective, a year's lagging behind on his PhD, a herniated disc, a depleted bank account, and a disabled little brother — not very results-friendly. But oh, from the heavenly perspective, so much, so much.

Last night, in our little fellowship hall, our church family gave Andrew a going-away reception, encouraging him and thanking him for the example of sacrificial love he had displayed to all of us. It was a close family time with tears and tender words, attending to something that had afforded us all a glimpse of our Lord Jesus Christ.

"God is not unjust; he will not forget your work and the love you have shown him as you have helped his people and continue to help them." Hebrews 6:10

Selah

I am speechless after reading this log today. Our hearts go out to your family. I am looking forward to meeting you. As a nurse, a care-giver myself to my elderly mom, and a Christian, I connect with your writing today. "It is to this you were called; to follow in his footsteps...." II Peter 2:23 – to follow in the footsteps of our Lord to the cross...

Mary Ellen Dove

Thank you for blessing us with a story of frail, very human humans plodding faithfully on. All of us must determine, with the gracious help of the Holy Spirit, to rivet our eyes on Jesus, the author and finisher of our

Chapter 13

faith. The alternative is despair, as life always fails to deliver what we had planned. And despair is not an acceptable alternative.

He who called us is faithful!
Leaning on the Everlasting Arms, with you,
Cheryl Nelson

In August, after Andrew had returned to Notre Dame, Peter's speech therapy really seemed to accelerate. He could tolerate the speech valve up to six hours at a time. And as the valve allowed air flow over the vocal chords, we often heard his voice.

The most exciting aspect of Peter's speech therapy was when he made his first attempts to form words with his speech valve on after some coaching from Beth. He said "mom" a few times, imitating her, and once when he was refusing some food he said "no" three times.

We asked the speech therapist, who was present at the time, "Is this early return of speech?"

"Yes, definitely," she replied. We called Andrew to tell him about it.

Pete also began moving his arms and hands more. His large motor movements were returning sooner than his fine motor skills. A couple of times a week the Lord provided a seven-person team to help Peter crawl during his physical therapy sessions. Occasionally we noticed he was trying to help with some of the work rather than relying on total manual support from us.

Another new motor skill Peter achieved was stretching his arms and legs when he woke up in the morning. Other than these things, he occasionally moved his arm or hand on command. When we ask him to give us a thumbs up, it was still kind of sketchy, but overall we hoped we saw it growing more consistent.

For months now, Peter had been able to recognize us and look at the correct people on command. He also improved with his ability to do this with objects, but tired fairly quickly, and would only do it during short periods of time. One of the therapists who worked with Peter was convinced he could read because he intermittently responded with his eyes to words written on flash cards, so we started implementing that into his therapy routine. It was still vague enough to leave some doubt.

Besides exerting his will by turning his head away from us, he also began to regain negative facial expressions. One therapist worked with him over a week-long period. She believed that Peter's higher cognitive functions, including long and short term memory, and the ability to read and make associations, were most likely still intact. She also used flash cards that displayed various emotions, and, Peter almost always looked at the "sad" flashcard. She said Peter is probably depressed, discouraged, and bored. This confirmed what we were thinking already, that Peter understood way more than he could show us. We tried to encourage him by mixing up the different therapy exercises to keep it interesting for him. We also read a lot of Scripture to him and encouraged him in the Lord.

Hope posted a new update:

Chapter 13

On Facebook:

August 19, 2011
Here are the things you can pray for:

1. *This Monday someone is coming to evaluate Peter, and if he passes their tests he will receive some state funding for rehab. If Peter doesn't pass, we will lose our chance at any funding for possibly a year or more. We know that God will provide in other ways if this falls through, but it sure would be encouraging to know that Peter was at a stage where he could officially receive rehab.*
2. *Pray that we would be creative in thinking of new ways to do therapy with Peter. This will help him keep interested and expand the range of things he can try to do.*

For the family,
Hope

September 5, 2011: What I Saw Was the Grace of God; A Message from Mom
I've been considering whether to post a story about Peter which includes some unflattering details about Doug and me. It's such a meaningful story, though, that I can't seem to get it out of my mind. It happened over three years ago when Peter was almost sixteen. Caleb had been nominated to receive an award at college, and parents were invited to participate in a luncheon honoring the nominees. Ours was a nine-hour trip from Texas to Tennessee, with a nine-hour return trip the following day.

Peter, Doug, and I made the trip—an easy one going up, with discussion and music and fellowship. Having his mom and dad all to himself was an unusual occurrence for Peter, whose three highly motivated and active older siblings often seemed to absorb all the parental attention. We laughed and joked and enjoyed our time with Peter. Once we were there, Caleb was grateful for his family's presence at the recognition luncheon.

The return trip home, however, turned out differently. Doug and I began to hear our Fort Worth duties calling our names, and the nine-hour drive home seemed eternal. Fatigue set in; we had been quite busy the week before we left and just wanted to get home.

At least I did. You see, even when fresh and happy, Doug and I have two very different philosophies when it comes to traveling. My aim is to arrive at the destination—home—as quickly as possible so we can get some real rest. This time my desire for my own pillow was overwhelming. Doug's way of dealing with fatigue is not to push or rush, but to enjoy the task at hand. And of course, being a normal married couple, we tend to caricature each other's ways. It seemed to me that he was stopping every hour (to get coffee, to take care of the side effects of the coffee, to get water, to get food). Indignant, I felt sure that food must be his god. When my turn at the wheel came, Doug found me a slave driver unwilling to slow down for the sake of anyone's comfort.

So at some point (I recall that it was while I was driving), Doug and I broke a time-honored rule in our home—the one about fighting in private and maintaining a united front before the children. We fought in front of Peter. Doug insisted that I pull over at the next exit, whatever it was, since I had passed up several beforehand in an effort to get more distance between us and Tennessee. So I did what he asked, and the exit happened

Chapter 13

to be at a bit of an armpit town in the middle of nowhere. The gas station was dirty, and the people in front of us wouldn't leave the pump even though they had finished getting gasoline ten minutes earlier.

At the Taco Bell where we stopped, the woman trainee who attended us didn't know how to use the cash register and was apologetically batting away flies while two teenage boys (the cooks?!) amused one another in the back kitchen, ostensibly wrapping tortillas. Their shenanigans conveyed utter customer disregard. You can imagine what all of this did to our already-frayed nerves. We now had something to be angry with other than each other! Peter watched quietly in the background as we slid down hill.

At some point, something happened to Doug. His strong sense of mercy for those less fortunate than himself called his attention to the harried cashier. He perceptibly softened, reassured her, paid for our burritos, and we all returned to the car. Once there, nerves still somewhat tense, he led us in prayer over our evening meal, "Lord, thank you for this food . . ."

Now if you had seen the food being prepared, I am sure the same thing would have happened to you: all three of us cracked up. We laughed and the tension melted away. We laughed until the tears ran. We laughed at the silly melodramas of life. And when we could catch our breaths, no one was angry any more.

Next time we stopped for gas, I was still appalled that Doug and I had tarnished our example to our youngest. I turned to Peter and said, "Peter, I am sorry you had to see your parents in a conflict like that."

Peter turned his ready smile to me, his shining eyes gracious and kind, and his voice very deliberate, "Mom, what I saw was the grace of God."

I have thought of this many times as we've gone through therapists who have had to figure out their approach for a patient who cannot speak, as we try to assess daily what Peter's capabilities are while he comes to new cognitive levels, and as he has so many people who are eager to be in on helping him. Some days I can imagine that we are frustrating him by too many demands. Other days, I am just as sure we must be boring him to tears, not stimulating him enough. When he looks back on this time, full of our ignorance and inadequacies revolving around his care, I am trusting that he will be able to say, "Mom, what I saw . . . was the grace of God."

Lord, preserve that spirit in him.

"I thank you, Father, because you have hidden these things from the wise and understanding and revealed them to little children." Matthew 11:25

Selah

All God's children, full of our ignorance and inadequacy, drown daily in the ocean of his grace. "Do you not know? Have you not heard? El Olam — the Everlasting God, the Lord, the Creator of the ends of the earth, does not become weary or tired. His understanding is inscrutable. He gives strength to the weary, and to him who lacks might he increases power . . . ." (Isaiah 40)

Grace. Everything is grace.
Lovingly,
Cheryl Nelson

Chapter 13

On Facebook:

September 9, 2011
Peter has been removed from the waiting list and approved for a rehab program. They felt that Pete was close to a Level 4 on the Rancho Scale, and improving. The trach will still need to be out before he can be admitted, so please keep praying that his trach can be removed as soon as possible. We are hoping for a short stint of therapy and assistance in removing the trach at Baylor before Peter goes to his longer-term rehab facility. Thank you for your prayers and we will keep you updated!

For the family,
Hope

Greetings,
Our family has been praying for Peter and your family since the Harris brothers first posted his situation on their website. We have joined in both your sorrow and joy. It is so interesting how you all have become a part of our lives through prayer — one of the wonders of being a part of the body of Christ. Just thought it was time to let you know that there is one more family up in northern Illinois keeping you all before the throne of grace.

With love in Christ,
Diana Navarro for all of us

Chapter 14

I believe like a child that suffering will be healed and made up for, that all the humiliating absurdity of human contradictions will vanish like a pitiful mirage, like the despicable fabrication of the impotent and infinitely small Euclidean mind of man, that in the world's finale, at the moment of eternal harmony, something so precious will come to pass that it will suffice for all hearts. —Fyodor Dostoevsky

Then, something happened that thwarted our plans for Peter's rehab for a long time. We took him to church one Sunday. He seemed fine. The next morning, however, he had a mild fever, though we couldn't tell that he had any other symptoms. Tuesday morning, he still had fever and his oxygen-saturation levels were dropping. His pulmonary doctor in Dallas offered to call in an antibiotic, but our nurse was concerned enough that she felt someone needed to see him that day. When his oxygen-saturation levels dropped to 90 percent, we all agreed he should probably make a trip to the emergency room.

That evening Peter was admitted to the hospital after the ER doctors determined that Peter had pneumonia. The doctors did a needle procedure, which drained a quart of fluid from Peter's left lung. He was immediately put on IV antibiotics. Though his oxygen saturation improved quickly, it was still low. He was closely monitored. We knew we would probably be at the hospital a few days minimum.

Hope's updates tell the story of those few days:

On Facebook:

September 28, 2011: Hospital Update
Peter's lungs have filled with fluid again and the doctors are looking at doing some sort of surgical procedure next. I think there are several options regarding what kind of procedure, but they haven't decided on one yet.

September 29, 2011
The doctors are going to do a procedure to scope Peter's lung. If they determine the pockets of infection are bad enough, the next step will be major surgery where they will have to go through Peter's chest wall. There is still a chance the antibiotics are doing their job, and that the scope won't turn up anything serious enough to warrant the surgery. Peter's fever is still high and his breathing is difficult, so he is definitely still struggling. Please be in prayer that the surgery can be avoided!

September 29, 2011
Last night the doctors put a drain in Peter's left lung. It seems to be working some, but they don't know how well or whether they will need to do something more drastic. The drain will be monitored closely throughout the day to see how it does.

Peter seems to be in a great deal of pain. It's hard to know the small ways we can help him since he can't talk to us.

Here are some things you can pray for:

1. *Pray that the Lord would encourage Peter and that we would also know how to encourage him.*
2. *Pray for our stamina as one of us will be at the hospital twenty-four, seven to care for Peter. Even though there are nurses at the hospital, we want to be there for him. Also, the nurses cannot hear when Peter's trach gets plugged, so it's important that someone is close by to suction Pete so he can breathe.*
3. *Pray that God would bring Peter through this quickly and heal him completely.*

Our hearts reach out to each of you, especially Peter, as we take you continually before the throne of Grace. May the God of all comfort overwhelm each of you with an awareness of his presence that sustains and strengthens you. Oh, dear Jesus, bless this family as only you can.

With love,
Diana Navarro

On Facebook:

September 30, 2011
The doctors have determined that the main pockets of infection are on the outside of Peter's lung, and that the bacteria is actually staph. Peter

Chapter 14

does still have pneumonia; he just has a staph infection as well, which caused the pneumonia. Now that they know what specific bacteria they are dealing with, the doctors have decided to hold off on the scoping procedure until the new antibiotics have had a couple of days to work. In addition to the antibiotics, we are keeping some hot compresses on his chest to see if that will help at all. Please keep praying that we can avoid any more surgical procedures!

God is big and so is his mercy. May it pour over all of you like an ocean.

Thanks, Hope. Lovingly,
Cheryl Nelson

During this time, my thoughts kept going back to heaven, and I remembered another of Peter's journal entries that had warmed my heart. It resurfaced now as personal encouragement from my son, as if he could still speak to me. This is what he would have said if he could. It was written two days after he turned sixteen, in his own humble, honest style:

It is Wednesday, August 13, 2008, but it has been a relatively boring day, even though I managed to write a poem. However, because of this fact, I will instead record the event of two days previous: August 11, which was my sixteenth birthday, and the day before, on which I celebrated an excellent sixteenth with my family. On August 11, I got to celebrate with my Scout troop. It was Monday, exactly five years ago, that I joined Scouts, and it has been an exciting ride ever since. I have learned hard lessons, made good friends, and reaped the rewards of hard work and grueling endurance.

But even more exciting than going to Boy Scouts on my birthday was spending a large part of the day in that which nourishes the mind and inspires the soul: reading. Rosie Watson, homeschool mom and co-founder of her speech/debate club, said "If you can't read, you can't write, and if you can't write, you might as well stop dreaming."

Why are reading, writing, and academics in general so important? It seems that our culture undervalues pure knowledge. It is important because God is a God of order, wisdom, and knowledge and because he has impressed a burning desire in our hearts for what is truly beautiful.

The book that I had such good fortune to finish was **The Brothers Karamazov** *by Fyodor Dostoevsky. I recommend it to all aspiring readers who would like to see un-euphemized descriptions of depravity, and unmollified condemnations of human nature in general, and who would like to have their hopes on one character's redemption raised to the heavens, then to see him turned around to journey in the right direction, though still encumbered by his sin nature (Dimitry).*

Life is no rose garden, as much as we would like for it to be. And life for the daily protagonist of heroic feats or mundane drudgery does not even end up a rose garden at the end of the day. As I finished **Brothers K** *in my bed at about 11:30 p.m., I gradually began to see that the end would leave a lot of things unanswered, unresolved, much like the discordant final note in the final track of* **The Village** *(M. Night Shyamalan movie), which I perhaps providentially was listening to as I read. Frankly, the last chapter left me feeling a little depressed.*

Chapter 14

I picked up my Bible and read Isaiah 26, one of my favorite chapters in all of the Bible, primarily because of verse 3: "You will keep him in perfect peace whose mind is stayed on you, because he trusts in you." But as I read on, a later verse grabbed my attention, one which in so many words, said, "Deliverance is not found on the Earth."

What? Are we really to believe that we shall end our lives without ultimate fulfillment, with loose ends still untied, with emptiness ahead? Not with emptiness ahead, certainly not!! No, instead, we look forward to the Final Culmination. We, as Isaiah 26 proclaims, trust that "your dead bones shall live!" We, like Kolya and Alyosha grieve the deaths of so many loved ones, but with them, we look forward to the glorious Resurrection: "O God, our help in ages past, our hope for years to come; Be Thou our guide while life shall last, and our eternal home."

God, our eternal home! Praise him and thank him for what he does on Earth, and what he will do at the end of all things!

Chapter Fifteen

So he had them into the slaughter house, where was a butcher killing a sheep. And behold, the sheep was quiet and took her death patiently. Then said the Interpreter, "You must learn of this sheep to suffer, and put up wrongs without murmurings and complaints. Behold how quietly she takes her death! And without objecting she suffereth her skin to be pulled over her ears. Your King doth call you his sheep."

—John Bunyan

I was almost thirty and pregnant with Beth when the doctor's report came back from my mom's surgery: she, who had baked whole wheat bread and made her family gourmet food from scratch every night for as long as I could remember, did indeed have breast cancer. A shock, really, to all of us, that even Wanda Weaver—beloved health food nut who'd welcomed one and all to her hospitable table and tried to convert friends and family throughout Dallas and Fort Worth to a healthier lifestyle—was not immune to the silent killer. I remember becoming nauseated, looking down on her thin form in the recovery room. She reacted to the news with disappointment, frowning and shaking her head. I had to sit down.

Chapter Fifteen

My mom kept up her warm hospitality all of the years she fought against cancer. At my parents' fiftieth wedding anniversary celebration—eighteen years after her first surgery—they received a letter from a good friend of mine describing the ministry of hospitality that my dad and mom had shown her over decades. The sentiments in her letter were echoed in dozens of other cards and messages referring to Mom's friendship and hospitality. A number of them made specific mention of her healthy, homemade chicken enchiladas and the other dishes she was known for:

I would never have guessed, when at eighteen or nineteen, I sat around your dinner table all those Saturday nights eating lentils and rice, that one day I'd have the privilege of joining in to celebrate your half century together, that I'd get to reminisce about the near thirty years that I have been welcome at your table and been able to welcome you at mine. . . .

Before you invited me into your home and family, I'd had no exposure to a Christian home of any sort, to Christian conversation, to righteousness taught and lived in a real, day-to-day existence. . . .

The things you talked about and the way you lived were foreign and scary and extremely appealing. Scary because they were of such a higher order than I was used to; I didn't feel worthy (and I wasn't). Appealing for the same reason. So I thank you for your true, lived faith, your open door, your open hearts, and your willingness to take risks with people for the Lord's sake. In no small measure because of you, I've come to know God's sovereignty, incredible patience, graciousness, goodness, and care.

Since those lentils and rice days, you've continued to show me such loving and selfless hospitality, continued to teach me through your lives and words about Christ, modeled Christ-centered marriage, and (Lee) mercilessly harassed me and blessed me with your (dare I say cornball?) jokes. That's another thing about you both that I appreciate—your quickness to laugh, to enjoy this life.

In the years following her cancer surgery, my mom attacked the diagnosis with pluck and austere discipline, reforming her already impeccable diet to radical proportions. Seventy percent of what she ate was fresh, raw foods. She avoided sugar and iceberg lettuce like they were poison. Between this and the Lord's good graces, she staved off chemotherapy and radiation treatment for eleven years. The grandkids grew up coming to her immaculate home, feasting upon the fare that this Gramma set before them, never aware that some grandparents loaded their second generation progeny down with candy and sodas. My children were in their teens before they discovered that snacks at other grandmothers' houses didn't include carrot slices, cashews, and jicama. (Their other grandmother was health conscious enough that they didn't recognize any big disparity). But, never doubting my mom's great love for them, they showed no sign of feeling deprived, or of not eagerly savoring the honey and carob brownies, the casseroles with the most cleverly tucked-in tofu, and the "treats" of raisins and cinnamoned apples.

Unsurprisingly, Peter, with his siblings and cousins, grew up genuinely loving carrot juice from an early age. Whenever going through various childhood illnesses, he meekly swigged down tumblers full of all manner of vegetable juice at Gramma's house. As he did, he learned of health and tasty food and trust in God.

In 2001, Mom was bitten by a spider out on the twenty-five acres of land to which she and my dad had retired to enjoy their winter years. She had taken out the trash one morning and had come back into the house feeling a sting. Soon she became white and faint. My dad called 911 when she lost consciousness. She struggled against the powerful toxin for several days. They decided that the culprit was probably a brown recluse. And for

Chapter Fifteen

some reason, shortly after the spider incident, her cancer returned with a vengeance. From that point on, nothing seemed to restrain its slow but relentless progression. Below, nine-year-old Peter speaks from a grandson's concern and faith the day before we heard the diagnosis.

September 27, 2001

Today is Thursday. I am going to write about Gramma Weaver. She might have cancer. She's going to have her test today so I gave her a get well card Wednesday night. It had a cartoon fish that I had drawn with my jell pens. I had copied it from one of my other jell pen drawings that was called "just swishing along." In the card it said, "Dear Gramma, I hope you get well soon. I am thankful for you as my Gramma. I hope you are encouraged by my letter." Then it said something else and then "I love you, love Peter." We are praying that Gramma does not have cancer. And I know that God will do what ever should be done even if it does not sound right to us, so I hope she trusts God.

During the last few years of my mom's fight with cancer, though she reluctantly agreed at length to radiation and some forms of chemotherapy, she never gave up on her healthy diet. As her body slowly succumbed, her spirit and resolve incredibly gained momentum. In the summer of 2009, she became confined to her home, and we helped her prepare the food she had once so eagerly served to others. Even in her confinement, she received almost three hundred visits from that August until she died the following February. People came to see her from every walk of life, from seminary professors to young moms and pastors' wives who looked to her as a role model.

Together, Peter and I (by this time all his siblings were in college) were frequent visitors to my mom's house that fall. On the chipped ivory keys of their old upright piano, Peter played Brahms and Rachmaninoff, plus some old hymns she loved, while my dad taught me the new blended diet he was feeding her—basically pureed salad.

One day I puttered around her living room doing a little straightening and dusting for her as she watched me from her many-pillowed perch in their cranberry leather recliner.

"Come here, Selah, and sit down, and let me tell you all that the Lord is teaching me."

"Okay, sure," I replied, and left off dusting to sit with her for a moment, not fully tuned in to what was on her heart just yet. My eyes flitted to examine the maple hearth and mantle with its white-painted filigreed inset which my mom had lovingly refinished years earlier. It had made a beautiful gathering place for the many who they'd invited to their home over the years. Was there still some dust over there on top?

Slowly she unfolded her thoughts for me. "Selah, when I was younger, I used to think there were things I could never handle. Cancer was one. I used to think I could never handle cancer, so I tried to have a healthy lifestyle, eating and exercising and so on. And then, twenty years ago, I was diagnosed with cancer." Her voice rose with emotion. "And the Lord helped me to face it and brought me through it."

"That's neat, Mom," I replied, beginning to focus. The autumn sun was dancing on the oak leaves outside their tall living room windows, forming a shimmering frame beyond her head.

"There's more," she said. "Then, I thought, well, okay, I've had cancer, but I could never face a recurrence. That would just be too hard." She slowly shook her head. "Then, as time went on, I did have a recurrence. And do you know what?"

Chapter Fifteen

I grunted the question.

"The Lord was there, and it was bearable." By this time, I knew that my mom was communicating something important to me. I was leaning in to her every word.

"Then, I hoped that I wouldn't die of cancer. I thought it would just be too painful, a really hard way to go. I believed that would be something I could never do." She paused and smiled at me, her eyes radiant. "And now, here I am, dying of cancer, and the Lord has been with me and is helping me to do it. You know, I understand that Scripture now in a new way: I really 'can do all things through him who gives me strength.'" Her voice joyfully underscored each word. I marveled at her peace. I felt close to my mom's heart, with a sudden awe of her that I'd not known before.

I called Peter to come back through the woods on my parents' property, on the other side of which he had been playing basketball in his cousins' driveway. Together we walked through crunching leaves back to our car to head home in the chilly fall air. As I walked beside my tall, promising son, I reflected on my mom's words. But how could I have known then the weight of the blessing she had just bestowed on me? How could I have predicted how her words would come to mind and grant me strength to walk this young son through the most tremendous suffering of almost any in our acquaintance a mere two years later? Her blessing, so deliberately and gently extended, would help answer our anguished questions about the pain that Peter would face during this hospital stay.

Peter's bout with pneumonia, fourteen months into his recovery from TBI, stretched the faith of us all. We felt so helpless as we watched Peter go through multiple surgeries those two weeks we were in the hospital. The doctors monitored his condition closely to see if it escalated enough for him to be put into

ICU. Later, we learned statistics that indicated that people with TBI, when they contract pneumonia, only have a 50-50 percent chance of survival, a fact that remained blessedly unknown to us as we watched constantly at his bedside. Hooked up to so many tubes and wires that we could barely reach through to touch anything but his arm, Pete could not tell us anything about where he hurt or how we could make him more comfortable.

Doug felt it hard one day. The doctors had decided to put a chest tube into Peter's pleural cavity to drain off more of the fluid they'd been unable to reach. They administered a local anesthetic and began cutting into his side and separating his ribs to insert the tube. Peter's eyes grew wide as he moved his crippled arms and legs around, unable to do anything effective about the pain he was feeling.

That afternoon I showed up to take a turn with Peter and relieve Doug to go out and attend to his pastoral duties. Doug told me later that he came home and cried and cried for the rest of the afternoon.

Hope kept all of the prayer warriors on Facebook and WordPress posted on Peter's condition. And I added my thoughts on it during a rare evening home from the hospital:

On Facebook:

October 2, 2011: Update
Peter is off oxygen and breathing more regularly now. His fever is coming and going, so it seems the antibiotics are starting to work and we are really thankful for that! However, Peter still has a lot of fluid in his lung, so please be praying that clears up. He still has the drain in, and we are

Chapter Fifteen

also using hot compresses and doing everything we can naturally to help draw the fluid out of his lung. Thank you for all your prayers!

October 3, 2011

The fluid on Peter's lung increased so much overnight that the doctors put in another drain this morning. Pete's fever is back up as well.

October 4, 2011

Peter continues to improve and the fluid is draining out of his chest. However, the doctors feel like there are still some pockets of infection that just won't go away unless they go after it. So tomorrow Pete is going in for the scoping procedure (technically a video-assisted thoracic surgery, or VAT). The doctors won't know if they will do a more major surgery until they begin the scoping procedure and see what exactly is going on. If they determine that things are bad enough, they will open Pete up right away. We are praying that the major surgery won't be necessary!

October 4, 2011

The doctors told us early this morning that they wouldn't be doing the VAT procedure today, but maybe tomorrow. They also said Pete's X-rays were looking better and Peter could probably come home a few days after the surgery.

October 5, 2011

The doctors said the surgery went well and that they were able to get all of the infection/fluid out. However, they did have to open Peter up from his back a little bit to get some fluid that wasn't accessible to the camera. The doctors said that they will leave the drain in for a few more days and then Pete will be able to come home.

October 6, 2011

Peter had a rough night last night. He is in a lot of pain because of the surgery and had a high fever and heart rate throughout the night. The doctors said some fever is to be expected after surgery but were a little concerned that it was high. Please pray that Peter will be able to heal quickly and that the infection won't settle back in. If all goes well, we may be able to bring Pete home between Saturday (at the very earliest) and next week. This would be great since Peter does much better at home and we could get back on track preparing for Pete to go to rehab. Thanks, friends!

Hope

October 6, 2011: A Far More Eternal Weight; A Message from Mom
A man undergoing heavy trial approached Doug for counseling recently. The man was fretful and downcast. Doug suggested to the man that he might be able to manage the burden of the trials more peaceably if he kept a noble eye focused on eternity and what the hope of heaven and the resurrection gives us. The man's reply surprised him: "Heaven!" the man snapped, "I don't need to think about heaven! I need some practical help for right here and now."

Of course, the whole point of Doug's pastoral counsel was that counting on heaven, according to the Scriptures, actually does give us practical help in our current struggles. We have hope that things will be set right, that faithfulness will be rewarded with the smile of the Lord, that earth does not have to be depended on to give us our final and settled happiness. We can wait patiently for it.

My son Peter knew this and believed it more dearly than some three times his age. With the many handicaps and setbacks he suffers right now, I draw comfort from his hope in the future. He settled it squarely last year when his godly grandma died. I recall keenly her last day on earth, she, sitting on the side of her bed with Peter's lean young arm around her shoulders, he, cradling her frail frame next to his chest as he read the passage below to her. Here is the short remembrance of that moment that he recounted during his grandmother's funeral last February of 2010. I found it recently on the hard drive of my computer. I hope the Lord will use these brief thoughts Peter spoke to encourage your heart toward heaven as much as it did mine when I discovered it: It was entitled "Gramma's Funeral."

"As a grandson I could give many dear memories of my Gramma, many examples of her gentleness, her faithfulness, her love, and her godly character. But one of my best memories of my Gramma is the last memory I have of her. I was blessed to be the last person to read Gramma the promises of God before she tasted their fulfillment in Heaven, which she is enjoying with her Lord right now.

"It was the day before she passed away, and my mom, my sister, and I had come down to visit her. I was sitting on her bed with her, and she asked me to read to her. Naturally, she wanted me to read the Psalms to her. The Psalms were always a favorite of Gramma's. She specifically asked me to read Psalm 71. It occurred to me as I read this Psalm to Gramma that not only do these verses reflect the power and mercy of our Lord, they also reflect the legacy of grace that Gramma left us. No wonder she liked the passage so well. She left us a legacy of a long life of faithfulness, joy in the word of God, perseverance under trials, and triumphant hope of resurrection in Christ. Those are the things that I remember Gramma for.

"Let me read verses 17-21 of Psalm 71, the ones I read for her that day before she died: 'God, from my youth you have taught me, and I still proclaim your wondrous deeds. So even to old age and gray hairs, O God, do not forsake me, until I proclaim your might to another generation, your power to all those to come. Your righteousness, O God, reaches the high heavens. You who have done great things, O God, who is like you? You who have made me see many troubles and calamities will revive me again. From the depths of the earth you will bring me up again. You will increase my greatness and comfort me again.' Psalm 71: 17-21

"I pray that the Lord will give me grace to live up to the faithful heritage that Gramma has left me."

Selah

October 7, 2011: Hospital update
Peter's lung has collapsed. The doctors aren't sure why, so they will be sticking a video camera down there at 1 p.m. to try and suction out whatever it is that is causing his lung to be that way. They have also put Pete on a more general antibiotic because Peter's fever is still high and they are concerned about that also. Please be in prayer for Peter's comfort and healing. He is in a lot of pain right now.

October 7, 2011
Peter came through his procedure this afternoon with no problems. However, his lung is still collapsed and the doctors are not sure why. He will be on a ventilator through the weekend to try to restart the lung. Continue to be in prayer for him. He has been in quite a bit of pain and is still struggling with a fever.

Chapter Fifteen

October 9, 2011

The doctors feel like the antibiotics have been working and Peter is doing much better. The bottom lobe of Pete's lung is still not working at full capacity yet, but the doctors say that it is not serious. They want to keep him in the hospital for a bit until his lung reaches full capacity, but we are all hoping that Pete won't be in the hospital much longer. The doctors still have Peter on the ventilator, but hope to take him off tomorrow. Thank you for your prayers, everyone!

October 10, 2011

Peter is looking a lot better today and is now off the ventilator. He is breathing very well and his oxygen-saturation levels are perfect. The doctors took the two chest drain tubes out as well. We are so thankful! It is rumored he will be released to go home in the next couple of days with one week's worth of antibiotics through a pic line, but we don't know for sure yet.

October 11, 2011

Peter is probably coming home tomorrow. I will update y'all soon on how you can pray for him about going to a rehab facility.

October 13, 2011

Peter is home! Moving him home wore him out. He had fever and dropping oxygen-saturation levels during the night and is pretty pale. The nurse put him on oxygen through the night. We pray that we can resume therapy soon and that this won't set him back in receiving the rehab funding. It is definitely going to take some time for Pete to recuperate after this ordeal! Please keep praying for his healing and comfort.

October 17, 2011
Peter is doing well at home. Although he is still very weak, he is getting better by the day. It is going to take him quite a while to regain his strength and responsiveness, and we would appreciate your prayers for his continued healing. Peter also has an upcoming appointment with a rehab specialist on October 25 (it was set before Peter went to the hospital). Please pray that would go well also. Thanks!

October 26, 2011
At Peter's appointment with the rehab doctor yesterday, we learned that because of the pneumonia, he had lost ground on being weaned off the trach. The doctor wants to wait a couple of months to ensure that Pete is fully recuperated and not at risk before attempting any aggressive rehab.

Peter continues to get stronger every day. We let him rest a lot because he is still recovering from being in the hospital, but there are times when he is very alert and doesn't seem to have lost the progress we made with him cognitively over the last few months!

Here are some things you can pray for:

1. *That Peter will stay healthy as we head into the winter months so that his rehab will not be delayed any further.*
2. *That the timing of his rehab will coincide with the time in his healing that will be most conducive to him gaining a lot from rehab help.*
3. *That the Lord would provide us with a wheelchair van. So far, every doctor's appointment that Peter has, he must be accompanied by Doug, who is the only one who can lift him into our suburban.*

For the family,
Hope

Chapter Fifteen

Over the next few months, this sickness would prove a big setback to Peter's recovery from TBI. The suffering he experienced grayed our heads and bruised our hearts. But, as with his Gramma, the Lord was there, and he helped us to do it.

Chapter Sixteen

Batter my heart, three-person'd God; for you As yet but knock; breathe, shine, and seek to mend; That I may rise, and stand, o'erthrow me, and bend Your force, to break, blow, burn, and make me new.
—John Donne

The November following Peter's hospital stay, Doug and Beth and I were totally wiped out. We had stayed with Pete around the clock for two weeks, Beth still trying to keep up in her classes and Doug still trying to keep up with pastoring duties— all the while waiting and watching intently to see if Peter would survive the countless infections, surgeries, and medications in his already-weakened condition. Then, when he returned home, we had to learn to administer antibiotics ourselves by pic line.

Peter's recuperation dragged along slowly once he returned home. In the light of our exhausted state, our church voted to give us a full month of vacation, two weeks more than usual. We were grateful; so many in our church family had shored us up over the past year of struggle for Peter's life. But because Peter's home-care was still intensive, Doug and I found it difficult to actually get away from home for more than a couple of days at a time. Yet

Chapter Sixteen

we managed to fit in several day-away dates during the month to enjoy the time away from pastoral duties.

During three of these dates, we wound up at Barnes and Noble, the rival to Half Price Books as our top date-night pick over twenty-eight years of marriage. On our way there, I voiced my discouragement to him.

"This is just so hard, Doug. I am not sure how much longer I can keep doing this." I leaned my head back against the headrest.

"We are waiting on the Lord, Selah," he reminded me for the umpteenth time. "You only need strength for the one day you are on."

"But what about Peter?" I wondered aloud, forgetting all my Christian answers. "Why does the Lord want our son to go through this great degree of suffering? He's such a good kid; he doesn't deserve this." My tired words of unbelief tumbled out, burdening Doug's already sagging shoulders.

"I don't know," he responded, "but I still find comfort in Deuteronomy 29. 'The secret things belong to God, but the things that are revealed belong to us and to our children that we might do them.' We just know what we are supposed to do. We don't have to know anything else." I could hear the strain of frustration in his voice.

My lack of sleep was taking away any ability to think calmly through these things. I began to feel guilty for weighing Doug down with my questions when he was tired too. Once we arrived at the bookstore, I said, "Look, you go on in. Take as long as you want. I'm just going to rest out here in the car—I'll be fine." He looked down at me dubiously, then decided to believe me and went in.

As he made his way heavily through the parked cars, I prayed, "Lord, please send something or someone to encourage him. Please undo any damage I just did to him." Then I tried to sleep.

About an hour later, Doug returned to the car. His step was brisk and he was smiling. I was so relieved.

"Selah," he began, "you will never guess who I ran into in the bookstore." He related how he had seen an old friend from twenty years back, now a pastor. His son, around Peter's age, had also recently sustained a head injury from a car accident, though not as serious as Peter's. His son was now walking and talking, but his personality had changed, and he had no short term memory. All of this had been very hard on his wife, the man had said. After facing the shock of the brain injury and going through the tedious recovery from it, she had quit going to church completely and was pressuring her husband to resign his pastorate. Her faith had been sorely rocked. Doug told this old friend our story as well and promised to pray for them. Though Doug didn't find a book he needed that day, the Lord provided something he needed more: fellowship with someone undergoing the same trial.

"So, you see, Selah, you are doing better than you think," he finished up. "Though it has been very hard, the Lord has kept your faith alive."

Since I had lacked the strength that night, I went back to the same store alone a few days later to purchase a few books as Christmas gifts for our kids.

As I checked out, I remembered Doug had a membership card which should entitle me to a discount. But I had forgotten to bring the card with me that day.

Chapter Sixteen

"My husband has our membership card," I told the woman at the register as she was ringing up my purchase. "Can I still get the discount?"

"Yes, what is the name on the card?"

"Doug Helms," I answered. But his name didn't show up in her system.

"What's your address?" she asked. "Maybe I can find it with that."

I gave it to her. When she typed it in, she found our membership.

"So you live on Wessex?" she said. I nodded. "I am your neighbor," she smiled. "I live a ways down the street from you. Helms . . . let's see, isn't Peter, the young man who had the car accident, your son?"

"Yes," I said, "I'm Pete's mom."

"We have been praying for Peter," she said.

That week, during our church family's Thanksgiving meal, Doug led us all, as he always does, in sharing testimonies of what the Lord has done for us that we are especially thankful for. Some thanked the Lord for provision of jobs during a lean year. Others thanked the Lord for Scripture that spoke to them during tough times. One thanked the Lord for his wife or children. Still another, for a family member's turning to the Lord.

When my turn came, I related the stories above as indications of the Lord's gentle providence in directing circumstances. A chance bumping into a friend we hadn't seen in years, who just happens to be going through the same rare trial as we were? A random encounter with a prayerful neighbor who also happened to be the checkout lady at the bookstore? No, these two meetings were carefully designed by God to remind Doug and me of his love for Peter and for us.

Two godly women in our church approached me at the close of the Thanksgiving service. Each was a member of one of our teams that come once a week to help with Peter's mat sessions.

One of them looked deeply into my eyes, "Selah," she said. "The Lord must surely love you a lot." She paused, tearing up. "Every week, I am just compelled to come help with Peter. Regardless of anything else going on in my life, the Lord compels me each week to make room in my schedule to come and help with Peter." She gave me a hug. "Surely, the Lord must love you."

Elaine, older and quieter, listened intently to our conversation. "Selah," she said, "you must put these things in your book."

On Facebook:

November 2011: Update
Peter is continuing to get stronger and we have been able to resume some of our regular therapy sessions with him. We are still working to wean Peter from his trach, but have received many conflicting opinions from his doctors as to how far the pneumonia set Peter back on getting his trach out and continuing with further rehabilitation. Pete is somewhat held up on getting into the rehab program until either his trach is out or he can communicate with us.

Please pray for these things, and please continue to pray that we find a wheelchair van. Peter's height has proved a challenge in finding the right vehicle.

For the family,
Hope

Chapter Sixteen

While Peter's home care and health issues claimed much of our time and focus, our larger life kept moving forward. For one thing, Caleb and Hope announced that the following May our first grandchild would arrive on the scene, God willing. This announcement generated no small excitement within the Helms clan.

Of course, the first order of business was for all the family to propose suitable names for the anticipated new arrival. The temptation proved quite irresistible. Soon-to-be Uncle Andrew, for example, eagerly threw "Thomas Aquinas" into the ring. As you might imagine, this offering drew an unenthusiastic reception from Andrew's less philosophic family members. "Caleb Junior," abbreviated to "CJ," was another popular label we tried on to see how it fit.

As Christians, we hoped that the names we gave our children would prove meaningful to them as they lived out their lives. Believers over the span of history have used the opportunity for naming to impart some spiritual blessing or quality or vision they have for their children. Little did Doug and I know as young parents nineteen years earlier how aptly Peter's name would fit him for this time in his life. Surely the Lord guided us to the name we chose for him, as well as to the words we spoke to him the night of his high school graduation, providentially ignorant of the way it would apply to his tragic struggle two months later. Here is the exhortation that Doug and I gave Peter that night in May 2010, inspired by the meaning of his name. We mean for the words to encourage him even more today:

Peter Douglas, The Name
"Peter, it gives your mother and I great joy today to celebrate the graduation and coming to young adulthood of our youngest son and child. You are the last fledgling to leave the nest of home, and so it is a bittersweet event for your middle-aged parents.

"Seventeen years ago, when you were born, our country faced startling challenges. Bill Clinton had just been elected, and we homeschoolers were apprehensive about what the change in administration would bring to our liberties and to our government. We wondered what his morals would bring to our culture.

"So we named you Peter Douglas. Peter means 'rock' and Douglas means 'out of dark waters.' We envisioned for your life one of those paintings of craggy boulders in the midst of crashing waves, the kind in which foamy green waves splash the canvas with ominous foreboding, while in the corner, large brown boulders meet the waves unmoved and unaffected, steady and solid.

"This has been our desire for your life, Peter, that when you see threatening waters swirl around your life, or the life of your country, when Clinton's plans seem paltry compared to what you may face in your future, you would bravely as the Scripture commands, 'Be steadfast, immovable, always abounding in the work of the Lord, knowing that in the Lord your labor is not in vain.'

"We have rejoiced already in the first years of your young life, Peter, as we see the Lord's hand on you, giving you grace to live up to your name. You have been, as one of your church family described you once, 'quiet, steady, and tenacious.' You have gone through challenges in the years

Chapter Sixteen

God has given you, and you have met them with a quiet fortitude. Mom and I remember that there were several years that on your birthday, you would end the day with a prayer that went something like, 'Lord, thank you for these (nine or ten and so on) good years you have given me, and if you are so good as to bless me with another year, I pray you'd help me live it for your glory.'

"You were on the right track here, Peter. You can't face life's storms without the Lord's help. Many times in the future, you will be reminded of your utter dependence on the Lord and on his merciful strength. Keep seeking his face to give you the steadiness to live for his glory when you feel you'd rather cave in, or you see others giving way around you.

"Remember that your 'hope is built on nothing less than Jesus' blood and righteousness. You dare not trust the sweetest frame but wholly lean on Jesus' name. When darkness seems to hide his face, rest on his unchanging grace. In every high and stormy gale, your anchor will hold within the veil. His oath, his covenant, his blood, will support you in the whelming flood. When all around your soul gives way, he still is all your hope and stay.' Christ is your Solid Rock, Peter. Stand firm on him."

Chapter Seventeen

. . . but I have prayed for you, [Simon] that your faith may not fail. And when you have turned again, strengthen your brothers. —Luke 22:32, The Lord Jesus, to Peter

Our dear friend, Betsy, from Pennsylvania, flew to Fort Worth for a week during the December holidays to help care for Pete and to help me achieve some holiday cheer. She and her husband were friends of Andrew's from his undergraduate years at Union. He had been Andrew's favorite professor. And Andrew had been violin teacher to their girls.

Her visit was well-received by all the members of Team Peter here in Fort Worth. Betsy wrapped presents, cooked for our family, did therapy with Peter, and prepared a care package to send to Andrew during finals week. She freed me up to design a t-shirt for those who had helped in our home, week in and week out, with Peter over the past year. We ended up ordering over sixty shirts—an eloquent testimony to the support God had so freely given us. She also helped me throw an engagement party for our daughter Beth and the young man who had proposed to her one chilly night in December. Betsy served hot chili and cornbread to Joshua's large

Chapter Seventeen

family and ours that night. (It looked like the Helms family would be adding two members in the year 2012.)

Betsy endeared herself to all of those around Peter by her willing spirit and her gentle and loving manner. Her service to our family would allow me to face the New Year with energy enough to plan a wedding and make ready for a grandbaby.

At the kitchen table one quieter day, she asked me what had been the hardest thing to deal with since Pete's accident. I could reply without hesitation: Peter had been eager and equipped to do battle in the culture wars Christians face today. Articulate and humble, Peter could present the Lord's case well and winsomely. Surely, as the Lord's servant, he would have lived an active life, zealous to be useful for the kingdom.

Why would the Lord sideline such a young man?

We were coming upon another holiday season without Peter's interaction. And following that, we would face another pro-life Sunday on which Peter was still and quiet and functioning at such a low level. Peter had always jumped into the battle for life. Over the days that turned 2011 into 2012, I kept thinking of all my young son had yearned to do for the kingdom.

I had often thought back to that conversation Doug and I had had with Pete over the Tea Party protesters. The father of one of Peter's best friends had asked him to paint a large sign on the trailer this man took to Tea Party demonstrations. This dad took equipment and helped set up rallies where concerned conservatives could speak and peacefully demonstrate. He wanted Pete to paint a Gadsden flag—a symbol of independence that flew during the American Revolution—about three by four feet. With the legend "Don't Tread On Me" already stenciled in, it fell to Peter to create the coiled rattlesnake above. After looking over a template, Peter proceeded to free-handedly sketch and paint a black and white rattler, the image of the one on the model, with one droll addition. If you look closely enough, you can discern a slight aberration: among the diamonds on the snake's skin is an elephant-shaped marking (not naturally occurring on any known Texas rattlesnake). Beyond the elephant's outstretched leg is an overturned donkey. The elephant was kicking tail, I guess—a display of Peter's subtle humor.

"But Mom," he had told me, "I still think Christians should be so much more eager to fight for the unborn than to fight over high taxes. How can we speak out more for the unborn?" These and other memories kept me awake at night.

So I told Betsy that day at the kitchen table how the Lord had comforted me, using others who had laid down their lives for the cause of Christ. I related my reflections on the Apostle Peter, who was told by the Lord Jesus that at the time of his death, people would dress him and take him where he did not want to go, to do what he did not want to do. Yet this was the chosen life and death by which he would glorify the Lord—not the way he would have chosen, but the way the Lord had chosen for him. I realized that we had to dress Peter and take him where he did not want to go. And this was the way God had chosen for Peter to glorify him.

I mentioned Lazarus, who had died because the Lord wouldn't come sooner in answer to his sisters' pleas. The Scriptures tell us overtly and astonishingly that the Lord delayed his help because of his love for the family. He *loved* Mary, Martha, and their ailing brother Lazarus—so he let Lazarus die. He had something he was going to do, and he wanted to let them be a part of it. He was going to use Lazarus' death as a tool to reveal something very important about himself. It was an honor, though a temporarily painful one, and one in which Lazarus was a pretty passive actor. Now perhaps the Lord would use Peter to show us all something about himself, even though Peter was a passive player in the action too.

On a particularly hard day over the holidays, when I was battling wild beasts such as would rival the Ephesian ones that Paul fought, I contacted Robertson McQuilkin for encouragement. Over twenty-five years earlier, Dr. McQuilkin had a thriving ministry at Columbia Bible College and was well known for his spiritual and practical leadership. He stepped down in 1990, taking early retirement in order to care for his wife, whose bout with Alzheimer's demanded his full attention. He chose to quietly care for her at home, for as long as the Lord gave him strength. So he labored, away from the public eye, for thirteen years, until she died.

In contrast, another conservative leader—a man whose name Christian decorum restrains me from putting into print (I am not yet godly enough to be able to attribute it to Christian charity), and who supposedly spent his life on the side of the Lord in these sanctity-of-life culture wars—recently said that a man may divorce his wife if she has Alzheimer's. Because the wife in question couldn't recognize her husband any more, this leader concluded she was no longer "there" and the husband was thus free to divorce her. After our journey with Peter, this attitude immediately struck us as morally repugnant.

In response to my letter to Dr. McQuilkin, I received a copy of the book he had written about his long experience caring for his wife. I highly recommend it—*A Promise Kept*. I feel pretty sure that, as capable a leader as he was at the college, Dr. McQuilkin will go down in church history not for manning his well-known position at Columbia, but as the husband who was willing to surrender all to care for a totally dependent wife (as the years wore on, she failed even to recognize him). He will be remembered as a Christian leader who embraced his pro-life stance with heart and deed. His wife's weakness afforded him the opportunity to show all of us younger Christians what it means to be thoroughly pro-life.

This man presents us a truth: the harder the task, the more heroic is he who prevails through the strength of the Lord. When I think of Peter, the Lord reminds me of Samson, who destroyed more of the Lord's enemies after he was handicapped and robbed of his virility than when he was young and strong.

I think of King David, whom the Lord preserved alive until he had served his purpose in his own generation. I think of Paul, of whom the Lord said, "I will show him how much he must suffer for my name's sake."

All of these dear people had their places in the Lord's cultural battles. And so does Peter.

So Peter still fights the Lord's battles, even if he never adds another word to those he's already spoken. His young life shouts its value. Sometimes medical people have told us that Peter is lucky to have a family like ours. If they knew better, they would know that we are the blessed ones to have a son like him. As he fights daily for his life and recovery, and we fight demons of sorrow and discouragement, we learn to be doers of the word and not speakers only. May Peter triumph more over the enemies of the Lord in his weakness than ever he could at full youthful strength! And may the Lord use his quiet life in the cause for sanctity of life.

On Facebook:

January 2012: Update
First, we are thanking the Lord that due to the generosity of the Lord's people, Peter now has a wheelchair van he fits in very comfortably. It has a fourteen-inch dropped floor and a ramp and CD player/radio, so that Pete can ride right beside Dad as he always has and listen to Michael Medved and Dennis Prager. It will now be so much easier to take him places. In the past, we were always dependent on Dad to do the one-man lift to get him in and out of the suburban. Now any of us can just roll him in, buckle him up, and take off.

Mom has been working on the book that so many have encouraged her to write about things we have learned through Peter's accident and recovery. In doing so, she has gone over many messages, posts, and notes that people have sent over the last year and some months. We continue to be very grateful for all that the Lord's people have done to encourage our hearts and strengthen our hands for taking care of Peter.

Prayer update on Peter and his recovery:

1. *Peter has been pretty responsive at various times over the last several days, now that the effects of the anesthesia and Benadryl have worn off. We seem to see him moving his arms on command, holding objects in his hands, and discriminating between the two by moving the one we ask him to manipulate at the time.*
2. *He also has been very attentive to conversation and reading from books at times. The other night during the family celebration, when Beth's new fiancé, Joshua, described the evening of his proposal to Beth, Peter's eyes were locked on Joshua the entire time.*

3. When we hold choices of books or movies in front of him, he continues to respond accurately most of the time we ask him to do things like "Look at the one that is a cartoon," or "Look at the movie that has Bob Cratchit as a character," or "Look at the one about a detective." We all think he enjoys those kinds of questions.

4. So far, Peter is still not ready for formal rehabilitation. Last week, he had a doctor's appointment during which the doctor said it will be more challenging than we originally thought to get the trach out because of where it was originally placed, and he has weakness in his throat that is causing it to collapse whenever he inhales. There are limited options of how to deal with this, some of which are potentially risky. There are other upper-airway issues as well. Please pray for wisdom and a way that Peter can be weaned off the trach. We will follow up on this in earnest after the holidays.

Hope

This is wonderful news—I am thankful for this answer from the Lord. Isaiah 40:31. You remain in my prayers constantly.

Blessings,
Bill Bishop

At the Arkansas tournament this past weekend, there was a girl new to our club drawing portraits of us competitors at the hotel. Someone had a made a remark. They said, "You know who else could draw that well?" and Ty Harding finished her sentence and said, "Peter Helms." Peter, even though I never knew you, my heart reaches out to you. I pray one day, I will meet you. I pray you will be in full recovery and you can enjoy your fellow "Speak-Outers."

Hannah Ralls

On Facebook:

February 1, 2012: Update
Peter is doing better after fending off a recent respiratory infection, but he still has a lot of congestion that we think is partially due to the all of the allergens in the air. Please continue to pray for healing and Pete's progression in therapy, removal of his trach, and for his speaking. Also be praying that an upcoming trial we are being given with a special computer would go well. It would allow Peter to communicate with us using his eyes to "type" out words or pictures. Thank you!

Throughout the spring months, the family was busy with the upcoming grand-baby, the approaching wedding, and Peter's four to six hours of therapy every day. We were grateful for everyone's faithfulness in praying for Peter even when the updates were sparse.

As far as his speech therapy went, Peter's progress slowed quite a bit after his pneumonia the previous October. We still labored to make it possible for his trach to be removed, but the process was tedious. From what we could tell, he made only intermittent attempts to speak after that. We tried to use an Eyemax computer to allow Peter to learn to communicate with his eyes.

That too, was difficult—computers always have glitches, and the muscle contractions associated with his brain injury made it a challenge for him to direct his eyes and head where he wanted them to go. One of the first times we were acquainting Peter with the keyboard feature of the program, I asked him to spell his name, slowly saying the letters "P" and "E" and waiting on him to find and lock his eyes on them. He was able to type "P-E", but the "T" was on the right side of the screen and it was hard for him to make his muscles obey his desire to turn that way. After trying it a while, we put the Eyemax computer on the back burner so as not to frustrate him.

In other therapy, we made a little more headway. For example, as we supported Pete's weight by putting his arms around our shoulders, he began taking occasional steps with his left leg. It grew stronger and stronger, but his right leg still pretty much hung limp, making it necessary for us to keep supporting most of his weight.

Peter regained half his smile, not as brilliant a smile as before his injury, but very satisfying to us nonetheless. It seemed that the cheek muscles and nerves torn in the accident made it difficult for him to use the right side of his face, but the left-sided smile he gave us was convincing. Pete smiled at Dad when he came in to pray with him at night, and he smiled during family hymn sings—always some of his favorite times when he could tell us so. And he smiled at Beth when she got in his face to cheerily bring him up to date on her wedding plans.

We sent out a prayer update in March:

Chapter Seventeen

On Facebook:

. . . In other prayer requests, we are losing two of our key players on "Team Peter," the group of people that helps us with his home care on a regular basis. Please pray that the Lord will continue to provide capable helpers that make it possible for us to keep him at home until he is ready for inpatient rehabilitation. At 6'4" and 170 pounds, he is pretty much a two-person job during the day, and a one-person job at night, when someone must stay awake with him.

We will try to get updates out more consistently. Please know that we are still very dependent on the Lord's grace for every moment and rely on your prayers as means of that grace.

Thank you, Hope. Congratulations on the baby and the wedding. And thanks to God for Peter's smile.

Cheryl Nelson

There was a lot of sickness in the family throughout March and April, but we thanked the Lord that Peter was spared from all of it.

He continued to make small improvements. His left hand began "coming back to life," and he could sometimes follow simple commands with that hand, like, "Peter, touch your ear" or "Peter, touch my nose." There were days when he could do this more effectively than others, but when he was very alert, he responded quickly.

Also, Rosemary began helping with his speech therapy during this time. She brought her violin along to play and sing to Peter; then she encouraged him to sing along. One time she sang "Holy, Holy, Holy" to Peter, then sang a verse with "la" in place of the words. She asked him to join her on that part, and he was able to sing one "la" syllable. She would also sing words to other hymns and leave a word out now and then to see if he could fill it in. We looked long and hard for this, but never saw it. He vocalized occasionally during this time, but no more than a sound at a time, sometimes the word "no."

I wrote a post in April to direct everyone's loving prayers:

On Facebook:

April 3, 2012
I will post some comments that Peter's Gramma Helms put on her personal Facebook wall a couple of weeks ago about Peter beginning to try to walk. We still mostly support his weight, but he is making early walking motions.

"Peter is so alert today. With help from cousin Daniel, he 'walked' from his room to the living room. He is able to lift his left foot and set it out in front of the other. The right leg needs help, but he was trying so hard to move it. After he was placed on the floor on a mat, I told him to turn his head toward the TV if he wanted to watch the basketball game, which he did without hesitation. Then with some coaching from Daniel he made two strong efforts to say 'no.' Also, he has some control over the left arm, lowering it slowly to the mat. Thanking God for his grace and love toward Peter and the family."

Chapter Seventeen

Continue to pray that the Lord will provide the manpower necessary to care for Peter in his home. The therapy every day in addition to care for his basic needs is daunting, and this past month, we have been less one helper and fighting sickness in the family.

His progress has been so slow, yet he continues to sometimes move forward by fractions of inches. Please keep praying for his forward progress. We still long to see a breakthrough, where he can make greater progress more quickly. Pray most of all that the Lord would sustain his spirit and our spirits as we day to day walk this path and that the Lord would be glorified in our midst.

Selah

Thanks for this update, Selah—from a mother's heart. May you, Doug, and family take courage as the months extend. Even so it is great to hear the small improvements in Peter's condition.
Stan and Elsa Whitman

Christ died and rose again so that no matter what our physical state in this life, we will dance together in the glory of our Lord in eternity. Praising God that Peter is a part of this.
Rachel Robinson

Thank you for the update. May the Lord bless you all as you persevere patiently in caring for Peter. I'm blessed by the progress (no matter how small it may seem at times) and the walk of faith the whole family is displaying through this trial. Y'all are an example of walking in trust and faith to the rest of us. Blessings!
Bill Heinrich

Peter and family, you are in my prayers this morning...may Our God grant his peace and love to you....this is not your ordinary trial...He knows you so well...
Jane Dawson

Chapter Eighteen

The prisoner, the sick person, the Christian in exile sees in the companionship of a fellow Christian a physical sign of the gracious presence of the triune God. Visitor and visited in loneliness recognize in each other the Christ who is present in the body; they receive and meet each other as one meets the Lord, in reverence, humility, and joy. They receive each other's benedictions as the benediction of the Lord Jesus Christ.
— Dietrich Bonhoeffer

"Ok, Selah, should I vacuum now?" Jane asked, her voice echoing off the empty living room walls.

My scattered brain manufactured some feeble response or other as the next volunteer approached needing guidance.

This was one of a dozen questions to which I had cobbled together a patchwork answer over the last hour. At that moment, around thirty folks from our church were engaged in happy flurry about my home—cleaning my kitchen; scraping, sweeping and vacuuming ancient carpet filth from my living room slab; improvising temporary spots for furniture in my garage; and digging around the foundation in our front yard.

"Where is Doug? Can we talk to him about uprooting this tree?" asked John, a young father in our church.

My fumbling responses couldn't do justice to the eager enthusiasm behind each smiling face. Every one of them had donated his Sunday afternoon to alleviate our newest crisis.

One of the many things you don't have time or mental energy for when you are caregiver to a needy loved one in your home is a Texas downpour. On the previous Wednesday afternoon following a late Tuesday night rain, our mat crew had arrived to help with Pete's physical therapy. Two of his cousins were getting Peter out of bed while I pulled the exercise mats out from under our couches. One of them looked moist. Had someone overturned a glass down there?

As we eased Peter down onto the mat, the knee of my sweats suddenly grew cold and wet as it touched the carpet. Oh great. This was much worse than a spilled glass of water. I stroked the carpet underneath the couch and realized with a sinking heart that, while we had been caring for Peter all day, our couch had been sitting in rainwater that had soaked through the crack between the wall and foundation of our house. It had seeped under our wall-to-wall bookshelves as well. The drainage route to our side yard had been overwhelmed by the volume of rain the night before; water had risen too high on our bricks.

I made it through mat session with a faithless attitude. After a hodgepodge of exercises for Peter — our minds weren't much on it — the guys began to help me unload the hundreds of theology and homeschool books on our shelves. Where would we put them amidst all the medical equipment? And why would God expect this of us on top of everything else we daily shouldered?

Chapter Eighteen

Next day, it seemed providential that Peter had a doctor's appointment in Dallas. Doug and Daniel took him, affording Rosemary, Beth, and me the hours we needed to rip out the wet carpet without endangering Peter's lungs. By the time Peter returned, we had air filters plowing through the dust- and fiber-filled atmosphere. Our living room was unusable for the rest of the week.

Our church family heard of the chaos.

My dear friend Jane often plays off Hillary Clinton's book title by saying, "It really takes a church, not a village." How true those words would become for us. The two or three hours that thirty people spent at our house on that Sunday afternoon saved us untold hours we did not have. By the time the men, women, and children of our little country church left us, our cement slab had been cleared of all furniture and prepared for new flooring. And within an hour after John asking me his tree question, he and several young men had rigged up a makeshift harness, attached it to the rear axle of his truck—parked temporarily in our front yard—and yanked the problem tree out from under our foundation by its roots. Brad, a structural engineer, had devised a plan to reroute our runoff water, and every book and piece of furniture that was still out of place inside the house looked surprisingly cozy, thanks to Katie, Lennie B, Michal, Elaine, Megan, Lori, Jane, and a host of teenage girls.

The following Tuesday, eight young men, ages twelve to eighteen—Nathan B., Nathan H., Robbie, Joel, Jim, Liam, Aiden, and Rueben—arrived to notch and glue wooden slats together to form a new living room floor. Under the supervision of Baker, who had taken a day and a half off work to oversee, they worked as hard as any grown men. Their free flowing banter did nothing to diminish their efficiency and did much to increase their joy in serving. And, though it was a skill they acquired that very day, they took righteous pride in the help they were giving us. Their faces glowed when we commented on how professional the job looked.

Besides all this, once the floor was settled, several showed up to move us back into our living room. Everything looked great, but I can't remember who was in on that part; so many helpers went to and fro.

Through the summer, our front yard drained properly but looked like Isengard after the Orcs had done it in—completely barren. Then our two Nathans (two of Peter's best friends from earlier posts), Robbie, and Joel combined their spare time to spend several evenings re-landscaping our front yard. They smoothed out the misplaced soil, laid a level stone easement and a decorative retaining wall, and planted a new tree and bushes. After dark, they would swing by Peter's room to say hello to him before they left. When they had done, our yard was presentable to the neighborhood once again. They expected no pay.

Their reward is in heaven.

This narrative gives only a glimpse of the many instances in which God illustrated his faithfulness to us through his people. A book this size cannot contain the countless times the same kinds of small miracles occurred, sparing us from being engulfed by sorrow and distress. Why did God expect us, on top of everything else, to go through our home being flooded? Because He'd already ordained his people to be his hands, feet, and heart in this trial. Why, indeed. The Lord loves on his suffering children through his children. The blessed result: not overwhelming stress, but sweet fellowship.

It surely does take a church.

Chapter Nineteen

When we shall come home and enter to the possession of our Brother's fair kingdom, and when our heads shall find the weight of the eternal crown of glory, and when we shall look back to pains and sufferings; then shall we see life and sorrow to be less than one step or stride from a prison to glory; and that our little inch of time-suffering is not worthy of our first night's welcome-home to heaven.
—Samuel Rutherford

Throughout the spring of 2012, Doug and I kept up a pretty good routine. Every Monday morning we worked out together—more a priority than ever for us now that long-haul stamina was so crucial to our survival. Amidst Beth's and my wedding planning and his pastoral duties, Mondays provided one of our few opportunities to connect.

During these dates, we often reminisced, taking time to grieve a little more at leisure. Doug was regularly visiting a young man in our church who'd been hospitalized across town for cancer treatment. When he did, he sometimes chose to eat at a barbecue joint where he and Peter had often eaten when they'd driven home on Monday nights from Peter's speech and debate club meetings, back during his senior year.

"Was it hard to be there?" I asked.

"No, it held good memories," he replied.

"It would be hard for me," I said. "Sometimes I feel like I lived the first fifty years of my life in a Jane Austen novel. It had its ups and downs, its joys and its sorrows, but it was a gentle story. This past year and a half, I've felt like I have been transported into a Shakespearean tragedy. Everything is so disconcerting and sometimes so sad."

"Selah, if you live in what our lives used to be, you will choke," Doug softly chided. "I know that I will eat again one day with Peter. Without a doubt. Even if I have to wait until heaven to do it."

Another Monday, we reminisced together about our past thirty years of marriage. I reflected on the highlights.

"I think my favorite years were when the kids were young," I said. "You were catechizing them, and while you were, I was learning so much doctrine myself. And when you taught it to them, I reinforced it in our life together at home. It was all so fresh and new to me. And they received it with so much eagerness. We were all learning how to enjoy the Lord together. Life in our home was like a little taste of heaven on earth."

"My favorite time is now," he said. "Because we see that they all adopted for their lives what we were hoping to instill in them then. Now we see the harvest of our efforts when they were young."

"I really like this age too," I agreed, "except for the sadness over Peter that won't go away." With Caleb happily married and Andrew and Beth both on the road to marriage, we had much to thank God for. Beth would unite with Joshua, whose goal was to preach and plant churches. And Andrew was on the verge of proposing to a girl who'd become a friend of ours while he was away at South Bend. They had met and formed an attachment to each other during the year he was here helping with Peter. She happened to be the daughter of Andrew's pastor during Andrew's years Texas A&M. All of our older kids were settling in to build intentional Christian homes with spouses who loved the Lord and were actively serving him and growing in their faith. I still so much missed all that Peter had once contributed to our family. Yet the Lord had given me grace: though tempted by my mother's heart to circle the wagons and pull all of my kids close to me during our family crisis with Peter, by faith, the Lord had enabled me to let them go. I knew he would use these new family members (including grandchildren) to enrich Peter's life.

"Selah, we have one foot in heaven right now. That's what Peter's situation has done for us. No matter how long we have to carry the sorrow of Peter's life, it will seem like only a few minutes once we reach heaven. So it's still better now."

Doug was right. We had a happy Christian home, made beautiful by the Word and the Savior. But, as our home rested here in this fallen world, it was subject to sorrow and tragedy. After all, it was only intended to be a faint picture of the real thing.

So I made it my aim to read books on heaven. I read one by John MacArthur and one by Randy Alcorn. I refined my imagination so that I could envision the solid stuff that the Bible reveals about heavenly places. Over the months, the Lord loosened my grip on this world and formed in me a new affection. I began to anticipate an eternal home, with all the warmth and love and joy and security of ours, plus so much more than I could dream.

I still struggled with joy, however. The only Scriptures I could hold to spoke of joy as something set before us. For the future. I still fought for a daily joy in the here and now.

Joy stole back in one day when the Lord pulled back a corner of the veil to show me how Peter would still wield a sword in his battles. The Lord was not finished with Peter.

I opened the door for our doctor friend one April afternoon. She had been making house calls on Peter since shortly after his accident. She came weekly to help realign and adjust the joints, bones, and muscles that Peter's accident had traumatized. She had become our good friend.

She asked if I had heard about what had happened two days earlier on the Dr. Phil show regarding euthanasia. I hadn't, but what she related horrified me. She asked if Doug and I might be willing to appear on a Glenn Beck show to represent a pro-life position. We immediately said we would. And suddenly Peter was back on the front lines, a soldier once again.

On Facebook:

April 28, 2012
The Helms family has a prayer request that has come about because of our journey alongside Peter this past year and a half.

We found out this week of a recently aired program on the Dr. Phil daytime TV show. The guest he hosted on his show was a mother of two severely disabled adult children. She was arguing for her right to decide to have them euthanized. Dr. Phil, as a cultural commentator, was open and sympathetic to her comments. At the end of the program, he asked for a show of hands of those who would support her right to do away with her children in this situation. The vast majority raised their hands. . . . You can find the program online.

Three days after this show aired, we were contacted by someone from Glenn Beck TV. Mr. Beck, a pro-life conservative, wants to do a program expressing the other side of the issue. He is gathering around twenty couples with disabled children to appear on his show and talk about the blessing that their children are, the sanctity of their children's lives, and their commitment to their children's care. We (Doug and Selah) were asked to be among the group interviewed for the recording of the show this coming Tuesday. It will air the following Friday.

So we ask you to pray for us, that we will be filled with the Spirit and speak that day for Christ, for life, and for the inherent beauty of a life such as Peter's. When he could talk, Peter himself was always zealous for the pro-life cause. May the Lord use him now as a silent spokesman to shout the value of life!

Doug and I thoroughly appreciated participating in the Glenn Beck show. We thought he handled the subject with clarity, force, dignity, and sensitivity. Many of the other parent participants were believers who helped set a faith-affirming and life-respecting tone for the interview. We were happy with the contributions we got to make as well. The Christian parents we met that day told many stories about their own pilgrimages with their disabled children who nonetheless lived lives of "meaning and purpose and dignity," as one father eloquently stated.

We met a sixty-ish mom who had parented her disabled son for thirty-four years. At three, he had sustained a brain trauma in a car accident and had subsequently made very little recovery. His father had left them early on. As a single mom, she had eventually had to institutionalize him. He was her only child.

"There are still days that it takes me more than one prayer before I can get out of bed in the morning," she told Doug and me. We marveled at her beauty and courage. "I still grieve for the son that would have been."

Now I am a practical gal, not much mysticism in me. But sometimes over the months since the accident, after encounters like this, I have felt like I heard the Lord himself asking me, "Selah, will you do this for me? Will you bear this for me?"

Two days after Beth's June wedding, Peter was admitted to Baylor with a goal of trach removal—the thing that so many had been praying for so many months. I posted a prayer update:

On Facebook:

July 9, 2012
To all of Peter's faithful prayer warriors:

Last week, Peter was admitted to the rehabilitation program of a Dallas hospital to focus on getting his trach out, with the goal of pursuing longer term rehab options.

While here, we have learned why he has faced so many obstacles preventing its removal, as well as so many associated problems that have made his respiratory care more difficult. The short explanation is that the trach was placed in the wrong position during his first operation a few days after his accident. During the original surgery, it was placed directly through cartilage in his trachea, destroying that part of the structure of his airway. Now the plastic trach tube has become, defacto, a part of the airway structure. Without it, his airway would collapse in on itself.

To correct this initial mistake, the Dallas doctor has recommended that Peter undergo a series of reconstructive surgeries to repair his airway, with the goal of eventual trach removal. We have been told that this procedure has only a 66 percent success rate due to the unpredictable nature of how cartilage repairs. (It has no blood supply and therefore heals very tenuously.)

This reconstructive surgery is a multi-step process that could take a few months. It could also be a very painful one, as the surgeon would remove a part of Peter's rib cartilage (causing the same pain as a broken rib) to graft into his trachea.

After much prayer and discussion with the doctor, we feel that Peter's longer term comfort, care, and health would be facilitated better with the proposed surgery. Peter has yet to progress far enough to make rehabilitative treatment effective. He can still do very little on a consistent basis.

Please pray:
1. *That the Lord will open up the way for Peter to get this surgery, and that the surgery won't set back his long term progress and recovery because of the weeks of recuperation and pain control.*
2. *That the surgery will allow Peter to regain more control of his upper airway, opening the possibility for him to speak and eat again if he continues to recover brain function.*

3. *That the surgery's rate of success would be determined by the Lord's favor, not the statistics expressed to us.*

Our hearts continually ache for Peter, who has endured so much suffering these past two years. A few nights ago, Doug reminded our children and me that God allows Christians to face all the same struggles and heartaches faced by others so that the world may clearly see the difference in the attitude of the response. He does not always protect us from suffering, but he always gives us grace to walk through it. If Peter has to suffer so much, please pray that he and his family will know the presence and sustaining power of the Lord in this arduous journey.

Selah

The doctor visited Peter at the end of his three-week stay. He had had second thoughts. He felt that the surgery might be too much to put Peter through, not knowing all that Peter was capable of understanding right now. He didn't want to put Peter into a decline, as he said, "I don't want to be standing around his bed a year from now, and all of us wishing that we hadn't gone ahead with the surgery."

Since the success rate with this surgery was not as high as he would like, he suggested that we consult with specialists in Boston and Cincinnati to see if they would recommend the surgery. We agreed to do so.

Peter's rehab doctor from Baylor arrived at his bedside the next day. She had a couple of assistants and therapists in tow. I could tell she wanted to talk.

"I want to let you know that we have never seen a family who has done as well by their loved one as you guys have," she said.

Chapter Nineteen

"With the time and therapy you have invested in Peter, you have given him every opportunity to make a recovery. Your family is phenomenal and your children are phenomenal.

"Nothing more could have been done for him that you have neglected," she went on. "And Peter has obviously profited from your efforts. There is no doubt that he is 'in there' and that he knows you and loves you and enjoys your attention. But he has not yet reached a level of consistent response that would rank him at a Level 4 on the Rancho Scale. Because of that, it might be better to delay the surgery until he does."

"There have been so many times we've thought this kid was on the verge of a Level 4," I offered.

She explained further. "Because we are two years out from the accident," she said, "the chances of Peter ever leaving the minimally conscious state have dropped dramatically. Usually, if someone is going to 'wake up,' they have done so by now. Statistically, he now has less than a 10 percent chance to ever progress beyond minimally conscious.

"But you shouldn't give up on Peter," she said. "You just never know."

At that point, I asked, "I have heard stories of people who've been in actual comas for five, ten, or twenty years, and they suddenly wake up and make a full recovery. Is that more or less likely with someone who's minimally conscious?"

"More likely," she answered. "And it can definitely still happen."

The speech therapist spoke up. "But it appears right now that you are looking at a long-term condition. And Peter is going to need you. We are recommending that you back off a bit on the intensive therapy, since it may not be doing him as much good this far into the process, and you definitely don't want to burn

249

yourselves out. You should continue to do enough therapy with him to leave the door open for him to come back," she encouraged.

"Peter is going to need you," she stressed again. "You must take care of yourselves for his sake. I don't know what your daily life looks like, but all of you need to keep a life outside of Pete. He would want you to do that."

"Oh, we do," I assured her. "Because he has as many caregivers as he does, we have all been able to maintain a life outside of Pete." It was true that we'd kept up pretty well with church, community, and family. Getting adequate rest and recuperation? Well, maybe not so much.

August 21, 2012
There is much to pass on to Peter's brothers and sisters in the Lord who have been praying for him these past two years. We need your prayers now more than ever.

We have received some rather bleak information in the past two or three weeks, since Peter returned home from Baylor.

1. *The update on his surgery: on the advice of the Dallas doctor, we consulted with specialists in Boston and in Cincinnati regarding the reconstruction to repair Peter's trachea. One specialist told us he would not recommend surgery for Peter right now because a patient must participate in his recovery from this very painful and extended series of surgeries. Since Peter is still unable to respond consistently to commands and cannot effectively communicate with us, the chances of success would not be high enough. The other specialist motioned us forward, but was*

> *unclear about the likely consequences to Peter's overall condition. So the two specialists disagreed. At this point, we are still praying about the decision, not wanting to rush ahead. We plan to talk more with the specialist who feels comfortable doing the surgery.*
> 2. *Peter's long term health care: another jarring note we heard this week was that the source of funding for Peter's in-home nursing care and doctors' visits will be severely curtailed when he turns twenty-one. He turned twenty last week, and will qualify for children's benefits for only one more year under this program.*

To give you an example of how this works, since Peter has a trach, someone has to be up with him all night long to suction the trach when he coughs. The manpower it takes to care for him all night long, and then to cover his nursing and therapy needs during the day, rings up to enough work for about four or five full-time people in a week.

We have always been wholly dependent on the Lord through this journey, from A to Z. Here is more to trust him with.

Please pray with us that the church universal can respond, not only to Peter's need, but to the needs of the many others throughout our country just like him. We would like to help raise awareness among Christians of the alarming crisis looming, given our current healthcare system. Our sanctity-of-life ethic is at stake.

And we ask you to pray not just for Peter's healing, but for sustaining grace during this walk with Peter. We need it every day. In John 9, in the account of the man born blind, the disciples ask Jesus, "Lord, who sinned, this man or his parents?" Jesus answered, "Neither, but this happened that the work of God might be displayed." In that man's life, the "work of God" was to glorify himself through healing.

In the apostle Paul's life, the "work of God" was to show his grace sufficient despite the thorn in Paul's flesh that the Lord refused to remove. His power was made perfect in weakness. Pray for Peter and the Helms family, that the Lord will similarly glorify himself by doing a work of sustaining grace in our lives to keep us joyful on our journey with Pete. God is worthy of our bearing this trial. Of course, we would still receive it gladly if the Lord chose to glorify himself by healing Pete as well.

Peter once eagerly desired to be active in the pro-life cause. As a mom, all I ever wanted was for my children to be useful for the kingdom. Perhaps Peter will serve as a compelling witness in the cause of Christ, and specifically in the sanctity-of-life cause. That is my ultimate desire: his usefulness to Christ.

Our son Caleb recently took a group of guys from his church to play paintball at a course operating south of Dallas. While there, they struck up a friendly conversation with the operator of the course. The young man thought that Caleb looked familiar. As they talked, the puzzle pieces fell together and the young man said, "Oh, I know your brother Peter. Our family still prays for him."

A few days later, Doug and I had a date night. We had to drive across town to find a theater playing the documentary that Doug wanted to see. When we walked into the theater, a couple motioned us up the aisle to sit beside them. These old friends we hadn't seen in a long time were there with two other couples from their church. They were all still busy praying for Peter, even these couples we'd never met.

Chapter Nineteen

The following Saturday was a tax-free holiday, and I slipped away to do some shopping at a local department store. In the store, a woman stepped in front of me and said, "Selah?" She also was a long-time acquaintance I hadn't seen in years. We visited for a moment, and she asked about Peter. She reminded me that her church still prays for him, and soon she volunteered to come help with Peter's mat sessions once a week. We had just lost our Monday mat crew, and she and her husband happened to have Mondays off—a perfect fit, a providential fit.

So we testify that in the heaviness of this journey with Peter, and as we learn to walk each day by faith, the Lord continues to send his encouragement, his comfort, his provision, and his people.

Selah

When Peter returned home from the Dallas hospital visit, Doug and I called a family meeting to relay to our kids, their spouses, Gramma, Grampa, Rosemary, and Daniel what we had learned at Baylor. It was a difficult meeting. After all, we had yearned and worked both individually and together to get our boy back. We'd hoped that by now he'd be laughing and talking amongst us as he always had before. We'd given it our best shot.

Doug led out. "Our family life has been rich in relationships all of our years," he began. "Our door has always been open, and our home has been filled with love and fellowship and laughter and song." He paused. "That must not stop. We need it, and Peter needs it."

He looked down at Winston. "We've got to have that little guy crawling around at Uncle Peter's knees. And we've got to have

AmyRose and Andrew, and Joshua and Beth conversing all around Pete, discussing the events of their lives.

"We need to rub shoulders with our church family, and have them here, and love on them here," he went on. "They need it from us, and we need it from them."

Andrew joined in. "Yes, Pete knows we're here and enjoys it when we just interact with him, without asking him to respond to anything. He still loves his family."

"And he always loved being with his church family," I added.

The previous week I had watched a documentary on Terry Schiavo narrated by Joni Eareckson Tada. I picked up a thread of thought I had heard on the show. "Peter is a person, who is living with a disability," I said. "He needs our love and support." This certainly was not our plan for Peter's life and how it would glorify the Lord, but through the laying down of his life as an eager college-bound Christian teenager, the Lord could still use him.

When Peter was about ten, we vacationed with some long-time family friends in the Rocky Mountains above Pitkin, Colorado. Upon retirement, the husband himself had built the majestic log cabin with tremendous windows looking down on the valley below. That week our kids coaxed hummingbirds to light on their fingers, played hymns on their instruments that echoed through the valley, and leapt over the rugged terrain with enthusiasm.

One morning, Doug, our three sons, and I resolved to hike up to the summit of Mt. Fairplay, a nearby peak that reached to about thirteen thousand feet. The boys scampered up the side of the mountain, while Doug and I, our lungs heaving, hauled our middle-aged bodies up the incline. The air was meager and the climb steep. Eventually Doug decided that he and the older boys had a good chance of making it to the top. Mom was more questionable.

Chapter Nineteen

And they really wanted to see the lookout shack that was reportedly at the summit.

Without thinking about what his youngest son might want, Doug assigned Pete the task of staying with Mom, while he, Andrew, and Caleb beat a faster pace to the top. Peter took on his assignment with a characteristic amiable smile, but I could tell he was disappointed. He looked over at me.

"Do you think you can make it to the top, Mom?" he asked, tentatively hopeful.

"I'm not sure Pete. I will try."

Together we set out; I had to stop every twenty feet or so to catch my breath. When I stopped, I scanned the trail above us. Even with the back and forth of them, switchback after steep switchback cut disappointingly little vertical sheer from the climb but multiplied the distance. Zigzagging upwards, it felt like we were scaling steep narrow stairs made of jagged rock.

Every time I stopped, Peter smiled at me. "You doing ok, Mom? I think you can make it." Every victory we won over the array of switchbacks immediately before us brought us within eyesight of a new collection, equally challenging, one right after another.

Peter was so patient and kind that at some point I asked the Lord, for Peter's sake, to help me make it to the summit. I didn't want to disappoint him. Whenever I caught my breath, I managed another twenty steps or so. Pete kept a steady lead of just a few steps.

"Come on, Mom, you're doing great," he'd say. Then he would glance up the vertical himself. I could see his yearning to be with his brothers and dad.

"Ok, Pete, I think I can walk some more," I panted, after each pause.

We made our way up the mountain in little spurts. His blue eyes kindled when it seemed I had committed myself past the point of no return.

After what seemed like an eternity, the climb leveled out, and Peter bounded over a shelf of rock that led to the ramshackle outpost where Doug and the older boys stood exclaiming over all the sights they could see. "We made it, Mom. Thanks!" came Pete's joyful shout, as he ran to join his brothers.

Truly, it had been worth the climb; we could see to the next range of mountains on three sides—greens closest by, blues beyond, and purples dim and distant. Having ascended to this great height, we gazed and gazed, lost to time, transfixed by the quiet majesty of it.

And so here we are, climbing a very steep mountain. I tire easily, and sometimes the way upward seems impossible. But Peter, with his usual patient affirmation, and just a few steps ahead of me, waits for *me* to make progress inch by inch. *Lord help me, for your sake and for Peter's sake, to reach the top.* With the Lord's help, we will press on, eager to join the company of our brothers. I hear it's worth the climb and that the view is spectacular.

Epilogue

If you would like to follow Peter's journey with us more closely, we post updates on his website

http://www.prayforpeter.com/

Here are a few recent updates from his blog.

To Peter's Prayer Team: March 11, 2013

Some of you have been asking for an update on Peter. It has taken a while to get one out as Doug and I were really behind on things when we returned home from Cincinnati, so thanks for your patience.

Peter is doing very well without the trach, though the doctors told us not to get rid of our trach supplies for two months, just to make sure that he can manage long term without it. We will return to Cincinnati at the beginning of May so that the doctor can scope his repair to check the status of its healing.

He does seem more comfortable without the trach. He sleeps better at night, and he seems much more relaxed in general. It makes me sad to think how uncomfortable he was for so long with that thing in the wrong position.

Also, the intensity level of his daily care has lightened significantly. It is less taxing to care for him without having to suction him every few minutes. Even though someone still has to be with him, the house is more peaceful.

Some have asked whether this means that Peter can now be admitted to formal rehab. The answer is a little complicated. The barrier that the trach presented to his getting rehabilitation is now removed, and we are so grateful. But in order for Peter to receive the most benefit from a program of rehabilitation, he would need to be able to improve daily on repeated skills. Because he is still so inconsistent on his daily responses, rehab would not profit him as much until he can build daily on learning new skills. We continue to hope that Peter will come to the point of readiness on his level of consciousness to receive inpatient rehab treatment.

In the meantime, we are receiving in-home speech therapy–building on the limited oral skills he has right now, like receiving small bites of pudding-consistency food and swallowing–as well as in-home physical therapy and some occupational therapy. More on this later.

When we cross paths with those of you near and far who ask about Peter, you cannot imagine how greatly you encourage our hearts to persevere. Thank you so much for sharing this journey with us.

Selah

A Good Friday update for Peter's prayer warriors: April 18, 2014

A number of people have contacted us recently to ask how Peter is doing and to encourage us to send out another update. Life stays pretty full juggling the pastorate, Peter's home health care and other responsibilities, but we still want to testify to God's faithfulness, as we anticipate celebrating this Sunday that He is risen indeed:

Peter's recovery has slowed markedly, but he has days when he is super alert, watches us closely and responds to therapy we attempt with them. His left hand remains trembly and imprecise, but continues to be his chief means of communication. If you hold an apple or banana before him, and ask him to take the apple, he will usually reach out and accomplish this, even though it may take him a while. We have tried moving from objects like these to letters and words, but still his responses to those kinds of requests are pretty sketchy. He is also very free to smile and hug friends who lean down to talk with him–he always seems to appreciate that.

For those of you who pray for us, we are asking the Lord to move us to a new home, which includes some sort of "mother-in-law" quarters. Our plan would be to rent out the extra room to a couple of college guys, bartering "rent" in exchange for a number of hours of Peter's care load. The last few months have been quite taxing to Doug, as he assumes the heavy part of Peter's care when others are not present in our home. So he works as a pastor all day most days, and then comes home at 5, when our caregivers usually get off, leaving Doug the lion's share of care from 5 pm-10 pm, when the night nurse arrives. It can make for draining days.

All this to say, that when we are drained, the Lord is very punctual in sending us encouragement, often in the form of someone letting us know of their prayers, and often in the form of someone offering to stay with Pete so we can go out, and often in the form of eternal perspective we get through the Word of God.

Peter's life dramatically differs than what we expected for our son, but we know his ultimate desire when he could speak was to be useful to the Lord. We do believe, though for the Lord's sake, Peter has been killed all the day long, and his young life regarded as a sheep to be slaughtered, (Romans 8:36ff) that the Lord makes his life an offering of useful service to Himself. Peter's journey with brain injury requires just as much or more emotional work as physical work, and daily we fight for joy. And we do it with these Romans 8 truths of the crucifixion and the Resurrection.

"Days of darkness still come o'er me,
"Sorrow's path I often tread,
"But the Savior still is with me,
"By His hand I'm safely led."
Trusting in the Wondrous Story,
Selah

Since Four Years Ago Today: July 29, 2014

We have learned that we cannot control what happens to us — we can only control our response to what happens to us.

We have learned to count on it, that on days when we are sure we can't take another step, when grief seems sure to overwhelm us and throw us off course, there is always prayer, sleep, and a fresh new beginning in the morning. So we don't get overwhelmed by being overwhelmed as much. (Lam. 3:22,23)

We have grown muscles to carry sorrow in one hand and joy in the other at the same time. (1Peter 1:7,8; Psalm 126:5,6)

We have been tutored in the summa cum laude of what the Lord requires of us: faithfulness — not success, not recognition, not

Epilogue

usefulness in a worldly sense, only faithfulness to the task He has given us. (Psalm 37:1-5)

We have come to know our best friends: faithful people who pray.

We have learned that in order for the Lord to prepare our souls for heaven, sometimes, all hell has to break loose in them first. (Psalm 119:71)

We have realized that the Lord reminds His people of stuff, and we don't have to fear being forgotten. (1 Samuel 12:23)

We have come to terms with that God's people don't always pick up on your deepest needs, but the Lord uses them to comfort you anyway. He's behind the human comfort they give. And even when it falls short, you are pulled towards Him then too.

We have learned not to judge people when they don't know what to say.

We have learned to move forward into peoples' lives, and not away from them, when our hearts are breaking.

We have been made aware that other people suffer. This is not always apparent to those who've not suffered.

We have felt God's grace sufficient. We once told people that God is sovereign and in control and loves you and can take you through any difficulty you have to face. But now when we say it, people believe us.

We have learned that, in sorrow, duties are gifts.

We have desired not to waste our tragedy, but to try hard to get the most spiritual benefit possible from it.

We look forward to heaven more. We know that when we get there, no matter how long Peter's suffering and our fatigue lasts, that when we reach that golden city, the ordeal will only seem to have lasted five minutes. Seeing Jesus will be worth everything. (2 Corinthians 4:17,18)

Our Thanksgiving: November, 2014

Last week, I had the privilege of speaking to a college class on the pro-life ethic applied to disability, age and illness. A student in the class asked me for ideas of how a person could come alongside a caregiver in a support role. Here are several of the ways folks have done this for us over the past four and a half years:

One woman packed my freezer with meals—one a week for an entire year: wow!

A man offered to get the oil changed in our cars.

Six women have faithfully cleaned our house for four years (two teams of two or three have come once every month).

Volunteers consistently help with mat session—Pete's physical therapy. We've had teams of three or four people for each day of the week who come once a week for an hour (3-4 pm) on their specified day to help stand Peter up, bounce him on the ball, stretch out his limbs, stand him in the standing frame, and so on. Several of these come from our church, but also from our larger Christian community. We especially need men for this particular activity, as it requires some lifting.

A teenage boy from our church volunteered on Thursdays from 8-5 (for a time) to come into our home and stay with Pete. He learned speech or occupational therapy exercises, so that his time with Peter was very productive.

A few people have learned to stay overnight with Peter. Men who are willing to do this are still able to get about 5 or 6 hours

Epilogue

of sleep during the night, while they take care of Peter's needs of turning, changing, giving nighttime water and meds.

A college girl mows our lawn. She also cooks supper one night a week for us.

Givers have contributed funds to an account that we use to pay people for respite and other extra care, to give us times away.

Faraway friends have written us notes and cards filled with Scripture, keeping us aware that they continually pray for us. They encourage us in the day-to-day perseverance required for a task such as this.

One college girl blessed me a lot by asking about Peter, his current needs and memories we have of him before the accident.

One woman from our church made cookies at Christmas in order for us to give to our neighbors—she helped us make a connection with our neighbors and night nursing help by giving us something to bless them with.

Friends nearby call me occasionally while they are at the grocery store, to see if they can pick up anything for me while they are shopping for themselves.

One of my children gives almost a month every summer to come and stay with us and take over Peter's care so that we can have one month of total break.

Doug's brother spends Wednesday evenings with Peter, so that we can both go to prayer meeting.

Eleven families pitched in for funds to buy us a wheel chair van three years ago early at the start of our care-giving journey.

A Christian businessman paid to hire one of Peter's cousins to work in our home 30 hours a week for three years back when he had a trach and his care was relentlessly intensive.

A Christian homeschooling couple (he was a doctor, she an occupational therapist) donated five days of their Christmas vacation to stay in our house and care for Pete to give us some respite time.

A Christian friend from Pennsylvania came for a week when Joshua and Beth were engaged, in order for me to get a head start on wedding planning.

One of Pete's brothers and one of his cousins trade out spending Friday nights with Pete, a night we don't have covered with paid help from insurance.

Our daughter in law keeps a blog going online, giving people updates on Peter's needs and asking folks to pray.

Girls from our church pop by sometimes and ask me what needs to be done around the house.

Finally, many people banded together through an online campaign our son Caleb got off the ground and contributed enough money for us to purchase a house that is much more accommodating to Peter's needs, a real treasure for him and for us.

So as this year comes to a close, we are grateful for the body of Christ, for how these of you mentioned above as well as many others have been the hands and feet of the Lord's ministry to Peter and to us. Those of you who would like to help: our biggest current need is for mat session crews. Contact us if you are interested in being a part of Team Pete.

Our Thanksgiving is rich indeed.

Epilogue

To Peter's faithful prayer warriors, news and updates — March, 2015:

So, the year of 2015 jumped off to a much better start than 2014 did. We are settled into our new home. It works very well for Peter's needs and for ours. Not only did the Lord answer our prayers for a more suitable home, but as well, he has provided already a young man to come live with us! (Remember this prayer request from last year?) Joe is a college student who also goes to our church, and he has been a good fit with us and Peter. Between this young man and three others that the Lord has sent into our lives–people who love Peter and care for him with a standard of excellence–Peter's needs are well-covered right now. This is such a provision to us, and I am so glad I have the time and space to write you how the Lord brought us through to this point.

Last year was somewhat discouraging, as we lost caregiver after caregiver over the months, and we had to pack up and move–always a major stressor–at the same time. I am not sure all that the Lord wants to teach us during those kinds of times, as it was super tiring and sparse in comfort. But I have learned that the greatest prayer the Lord can answer on our behalf is to keep us faithful unto death. James 5:11 tells us that we can consider a person blessed by the Lord when he remains faithful under trial. The same sentiment shows up in Psalm 119:56, which indicates the Lord's blessing on a person sparkles, not when everything is going well, but when he obeys the Lord's precepts faithfully.

It appears evident the Scripture views faithfulness as the big catch, not freedom from being inconvenienced, or freedom from pain and suffering, or even freedom to have an easy time of doing what we think God wants us to do. How we have been blessed if the Lord keeps us faithfully on the path, doggedly so, in spite of setbacks and hardships!

Now that these provisions are in place, we don't put our hope in them, but in the Lord's faithfulness to us to keep us faithful in plenty or in want. However, I am hopeful that I will have more opportunities to write for this blog, because there are other things I think the Lord is giving to us that I want to share. So, more soon, Lord willing.

Learning to live to hear the "well-done,"

Selah (for Doug, Peter, and the family)

Appendix A

August 16, 2010: Message from Mom

Sunday morning, in Peter's Bible again (NKJV), from the book of Jeremiah, with his comments in brackets following the quoted verses. Parentheticals mine:

> "'They do not plead the cause, the cause of the fatherless; Yet they prosper, And the right of the needy they do not defend. Shall I not punish them for these things?' says the Lord." — Jeremiah 5:28 [We are called to willingly give charity. Without active charity, a nation will be judged.]

> "An astonishing and horrible thing has been committed in the land: The prophets prophesy falsely, and the priests rule by their own power; And My people love to have it so. But what will you do in the end?" — Jeremiah 5:30-31 [Eternity always convicts. Vanity, all is vanity.]

> "'And like their bow they have bent their tongues for lies. They are not valiant for the truth on the earth. For they proceed

from evil to evil, and they do not know Me,' says the Lord." — Jeremiah 9:3 *[Not being valiant for truth is a sign of not knowing God as much as we ought.]*

"Therefore a lion from the forest shall slay them, A wolf of the deserts shall destroy them; A leopard shall watch over their cities." — Jeremiah 5:6 *[Dante's Inferno (Peter read this for school).]*

"And it shall come to pass at that time, that I will search Jerusalem with lamps, and punish the men who are settled in complacency, who say in their heart, 'The Lord will not do good, nor will He do evil.'" — Zephaniah 1:12 *[Deism: "God does not act."]*

"Seek the Lord, all you meek of the earth, who have upheld His justice. Seek righteousness, seek humility. It may be that you will be hidden in the day of the Lord's anger." — Zephaniah 2:3 *[Message of hope — hidden in Christ.]*

"For then I will restore to the peoples a pure language . . .[The curse is reversed in the Kingdom.]. . .that they all may call on name of the Lord, to serve Him with one accord." — Zephaniah 3:9 *[With one accord means shoulder to shoulder.]*

" . . . The daughters of My dispersed ones, shall bring My offering. In that day you shall not be shamed for any of your deeds in which you transgress against Me." — Zephaniah 3:10,11a (capitalized personal pronouns underlined) *[The Emphasis is on God.]*

Appendix A

"The Lord your God in your midst, The Mighty One, will save; He will rejoice over you with gladness, He will quiet you with His love, He will rejoice over you with singing." —Zephaniah 3:17 [The Lamb is all the glory in Immanuel's land (line from one of Peter's favorite hymns: "The Sands of Time are Sinking"). Message of hope.]

Selah

August 23, 2010: Notes from Pete's Bible
Sunday morning in New Testament Letters with Pete, his comments in brackets beside the underlined verses. Parentheticals mine:

"I have been crucified with Christ; it is no longer I who live, but Christ lives in me; and the life which I now live in the flesh I live by faith in the Son of God, who loved me and gave Himself for me." —Galatians 2:20 (the word "me" is underlined) [Christ died for individuals.]

"For you were once darkness, but now you are light in the Lord. Walk as children of light, for the fruit of the Spirit is in all goodness, righteousness, and truth, finding out what is acceptable to the Lord." —Ephesians 5:8-10 [We want to walk in the light because God has saved us from the realm of death.]

" . . . be filled with the Spirit, speaking to one another in psalms and hymns and spiritual songs, singing and making melody in your heart to the Lord, giving thanks always for all things to God the Father in the name of our Lord Jesus Christ, submitting

to one another in the fear of God." —Ephesians 5:18-21 [Outdo each other in serving one another. Submit to everyone in love. This does not teach egalitarianism.]

"For though by this time you ought to be teachers, you need someone to teach you again the first principles of the oracles of God, and you have come to need milk and not solid food." —Hebrews 5:12 [Spiritual backsliding.]

"But solid food belongs to those who are of full age, that is, those who by reason of use have their senses exercised to discern both good and evil." —Hebrews 5:14 [Senses of discernment—we must use them and exercise them by the Spirit.]

"My son, do not despise the chastening of the Lord, nor be discouraged when you are rebuked by Him; for whom the Lord loves He chastens, and scourges every son whom He receives." —Hebrews 12:6 [When you face trials, remember Christ is treating you as a son.]

September 14, 2010: From Peter's Bible
From Peter's Bible again, through the book of James:

"My brethren, count it all joy when you fall into various trials, knowing that the testing of your faith produces patience." —James 1:2, 3 [Sanctification through hardship.]

"Let the lowly brother glory in his exaltation, but the rich in his humiliation . . ." —James 1:9 [Rich in Christ.]

Appendix A

"Blessed is the man who endures temptation; for when he has been approved, he will receive the crown of life, which the Lord has promised to those who love Him." — James 1:12 [God gives and approves the tests. God does not tempt.]

"Of His own will He brought us forth by the word of truth, that we might be a kind of firstfruits of His creatures." — James 1:18 [Man is God's creative masterpiece.]

"Therefore lay aside all filthiness and overflow of wickedness, and receive with meekness the implanted word, which is able to save your souls. But be doers of the word, and not hearers only . . ." — James 1:21, 22 [Receive with meekness and do it.]

"But he who looks into the perfect law of liberty and continues in it, and is not a forgetful hearer, but a doer of the work, this one will be blessed in what he does." — James 1:25 [Continue diligently in the Word; it is the law of life and liberty.]

"If anyone among you thinks he is religious, and does not bridle his tongue, but deceives his own heart, this one's religion is useless. Pure and undefiled religion before God and the Father is this: to visit orphans and widows in their trouble, and to keep oneself unspotted from the world." — James 1:26, 27 [Faith shows itself through works.]

"Where do wars and fights come from among you? Do they not come from your desires for pleasure that war in your members? You lust and do not have." — James 4:1, 2 [Self-centeredness.

The world, the flesh, and the devil, yet you are always responsible for your sin.]

"You ask and do not receive, because you ask amiss, that you may spend it on your pleasures. Adulterers and adulteresses! Do you not know that friendship with the world is enmity with God?"
—James 4:3, 4 [Unfaithful to covenant relationship.]

Appendix B

Re: National Merit Recommendation for Peter Helms
To whom it may concern:

Peter Helms is a person who has constantly surprised me over the past several years, particularly in the classroom. (I've taught him literature, history, and government.) The surprise comes from Peter's being so unassuming, yet so capable. Here's a young man who's failed to pick up the habits of his culture. For example, Peter seems to have no expectation that others should admire or defer to him. Indeed, he's quick to accept duties that are unglamorous, even anonymous. He rarely draws attention to himself, but neither does he shun attention when he can thereby help move the ball forward (*whatever* that ball may be). He respects authority because it's his duty to respect and assist those in positions over him, and also because he recognizes that authority generally knows more and better than he does.

But Peter surprises more by what he is than what he is not. His unassuming ways reflect no lack of confidence. Rather, Peter is always watching, always considering. And his curiosity is both wondrous and compassionate. He's able to sense the ways in which those around him are struggling, and he cares. Perhaps it's because of these practices and attitudes that others often choose Peter to lead. He's the one who both the adults and the other kids know will get the job done, and done gracefully. When he occasionally volunteers himself, it's out of duty rather than ego. Because Peter is a servant leader, others single him out as the one they will follow.

Peter also excels as a thinker. My classes in western civilization include strong secondary emphasis on philosophy/thought. In these classes, Peter has been required to read a good number of the classics in literature and philosophy, to write on them and discuss their merits in class, and occasionally even to perform them publically. I will not soon forget the impressive oratory skills Peter surprised us with during his portrayal of Mark Antony in a production of Julius Caesar when Peter was in ninth grade.

This classical education has brought out and developed Peter's affinity for most all of the humanities, and it has helped inflame his curiosity about our own day: Who should lead? Why? How should they lead? What values are universal? Why do some people see this otherwise? Have we learned from history? What *should* we learn? How do we know what is true? Yes, these types of questions have come up in Peter's reading of Homer (the *Odyssey*), Plato (the *Republic*), Aristotle (*Poetics*), Sophocles (*Antigone*), Virgil (the *Aeneid*), Livy, Augustine (*Confessions*), Dante (*Inferno*), Shakespeare (*Henry V, Macbeth*), Luther, Calvin, Madison, Paine, Burke, Tocqueville, Marx (*Communist Manifesto*), Freud, and so on. What I've noticed about Peter's study is his quick grasp and assimilation of these thinkers into his own expanding worldview. He catches what they're saying, within the context of their times, and he lets them influence him in all the ways they should.

Intellectually, Peter is becoming a smart realist about the world in which he lives. But he shows no signs of the cynicism or sardonic criticism that characterize so many who follow the events of our day. Finally, Peter is a learner, an observer, a reader, and a thinker in a world full of young people who are busy blogging, twittering, and posting their every movement and random thought for posterity. Twenty years from now, no one will tarnish Peter's contributions by trotting out any embarrassing paragraphs that he shot off during his youth.

For all of this, Peter isn't really bookish. Although he's an outstanding student whom I would label a real thinker in a way that few are, he's more about action. Peter is an artist, a writer, a speaker, debater (competitive), leader, Boy Scout, and frequent community volunteer. He's not in love with learning for its own sake so much, I think, as for the sake of what he's going to do with it, how he's going to impact the world as a fully educated person. But that doesn't quite capture what he's about either, because I don't believe Peter looks on knowledge as a tool. Rather, knowledge is inspiring him toward action. He seems to feel an urgency to get to a point at which he can really do some good with it. I'm eager to see what that good turns out to be.

Even among the many outstanding homeschooled students I've taught over the last few years, Peter has consistently surprised me with his ability, dependability, and the keen, gracious insights he gleans from watching and being ready to serve.

I recommend him for the highest scholarship available at any academic institution.

Sincerely,
Susan Kahler
J.D., B.S. (Journalism)

Endorsements

That Your Faith May Not Fail is a poignant and moving account of God's faithfulness in the midst of great challenge and serious struggle. In an inspiring and profoundly stirring way, Selah Helms offers great wisdom and guidance to help us in the midst of life's most difficult setbacks, those times of deep suffering and pain. Highly recommended!
David S. Dockery, Ph.D
President, Trinity International University

That Your Faith May Not Fail: Peter's Sermon is a book about many things: a son who loved the Lord and was a blessing to be around before and after his tragic accident, the precious sanctity of life, the sustained grace of God, the hope of heaven, the prayers of a myriad of saints, many medical and lay people with merciful and servant's hearts, Providential witnessing opportunities, grief, and perseverance. But most of all, this book is about a high view of God — His sovereignty, His love, and His kindness throughout devastating circumstances.

Endorsements

Selah Helms is a faithful pastor's wife and homeschool Mom. She has written a captivating book that I could hardly put down. The story is gripping and God-honoring as Selah and her husband Doug and their children grapple with the events of Peter's accident and afterwards. Children are, most certainly, a blessing from God. Peter was such a blessing even as a little child and even after his devastating accident. This is one book you will want to read. I highly recommend it.

Martha Peace,
Biblical Counselor and author of *The Excellent Wife*

It has been a rich blessing for me and my family to know and love the Helms family. Since we first met their older two sons when they came to Union, the Helms became dear friends and helpful examples to us.

This moving account of how they have and are walking through the ordeal of Peter's suffering is truly powerful. I was challenged and encouraged by reading it. I found myself yearning to know God more richly, to trust Him more fully, to love my family more deeply, and to immerse myself more completely into God's Word. I urge you to read this book and pass it on to others because it will be useful in building up believers and calling people to faith in Jesus, as it recounts how this family has found God faithful as they have been held fast by the great gospel truths.

Ray Van Neste, Ph.D,
Director of the R.C. Ryan Center for Biblical Studies and Professor of Biblical studies, Union University

As a certified Family and Consumer Scientist whose life's vocation and ministry is focused on training women to joyfully assume their God mandated role in the home, church, and community, I am pleased to recommend That Your Faith May not Fail, Peter's Sermon. This resource will stimulate the reader to view the sanctity of life through the lens of scripture concurrently with providing practical helps for any woman to assume the biblical role of caregiver. Knowing the Helms family personally, I can affirm that they daily model their trust in their heavenly Father and His sovereignty that the book so clearly presents regardless of the outward circumstances.

Patricia A. Ennis, Ph. D, CFCS
Distinguished Professor of Homemaking and Director of Homemaking Programs,
Southwestern Baptist Theological Seminary

I am abundantly grateful to the LORD for the inspiring privilege to read *That Your Faith May Not Fail: Peter's Sermon*. It has caused me yet again to be thankful for the depth of our belief system and the Holy Spirit's empowerment to help us live out what we say we believe. Of any worldview Christianity speaks profoundly about how to view suffering. After all, a cross is the central emblem of our theology!

In the midst of a culture that speaks of "quality of life" issues and devalues suffering, the Helms' God-given testimony speaks like a megaphone. Our belief system tells us that Peter has been used of the LORD to teach others to sacrificially love. In the midst of skepticism about the value of the Church he has been used by our LORD to show the beauty of the body of Christ in action. In the midst of the degradation of the American family, He has allowed the Helms family to model its tremendous depth and beauty. Please feed your soul and reinforce your theology by reading this book.

Ernie Baker, D.Min

Professor of Biblical Counseling

The Master's College

Fellow, The Association of Certified Biblical Counselors

Author of *Help! I'm in a Conflict and Marry Wisely, Marry Well* (Shepherd Press)

About the author:

Selah Helms has supported her husband Doug's pastoral ministry for twenty years, while raising four children. She teaches Western Civilization to homeschoolers, speaks on discipling children, and co-authored the two volumes of *Small Talks on Big Questions,* a historical companion to the children's catechism (based on the Spurgeon's Baptist Catechism).